PLANT-BASED DIET COOKBOOK FOR SENIORS

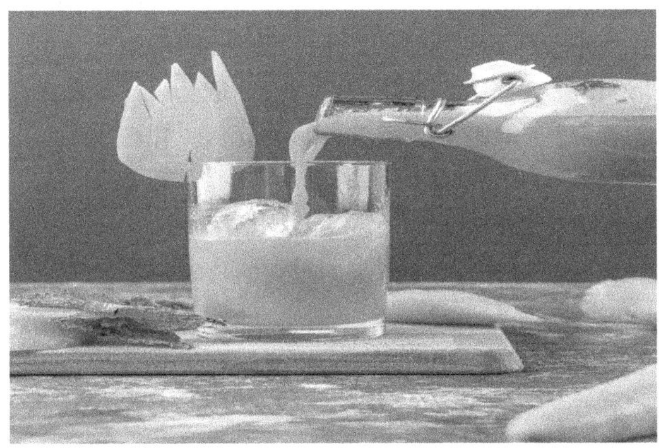

A Culinary Guide To Overcoming Low Libido With Refreshing & Nourishing Recipes For Sexual Wellness

Ericson Carpenter

TABLE OF CONTENT

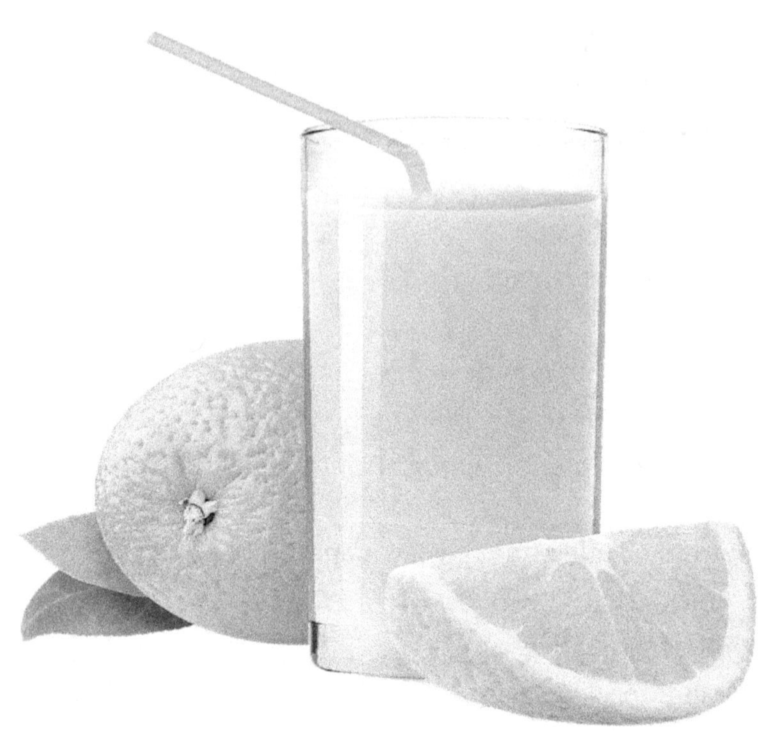

INTRODUCTION

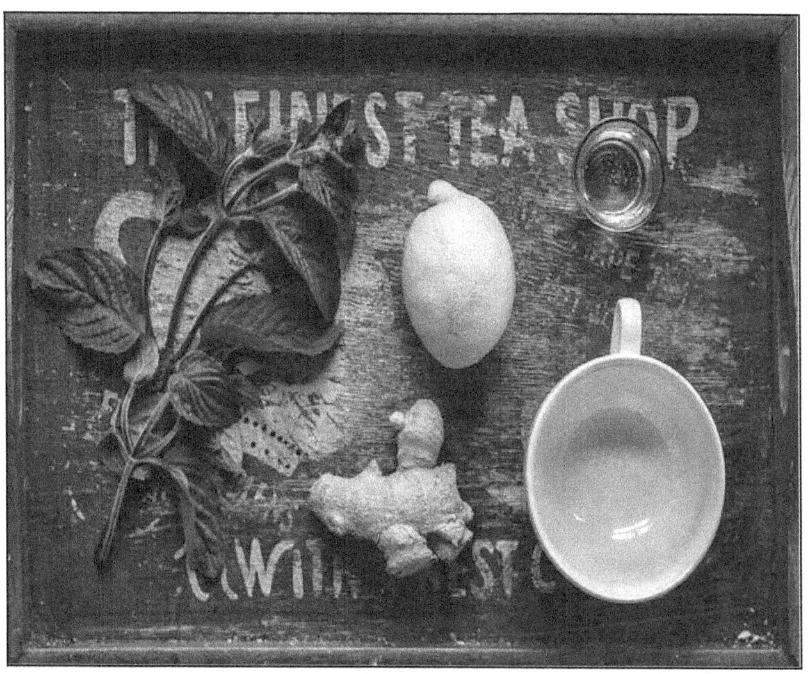

Welcome to Men's Health Plant-based Diet Cookbook for seniors. In the modern world, where a multitude of factors can impact men's health, it's essential to explore holistic approaches to enhance well-being. This culinary guide delves into the intersection of nutrition and men's sexual health, harnessing the power of plant-based ingredients to support vitality, stamina, and overall sexual wellness. In a society where fast-paced lifestyles and stressors abound, it's crucial to adopt a proactive and sustainable approach to maintaining one's health. Rather than relying solely on conventional solutions,this guide advocates for the incorporation of nutrient-rich, plant-based foods into your daily diet. By making mindful choices in the kitchen, you can embark on a journey toward optimizing your sexual wellness while savoring delicious and nourishing meals. Within these pages, we'll explore a diverse array of plant-powered ingredients,each chosen for its potential to boost libido, improve circulation, and contribute to hormonal balance. From nutrient-dense fruits and vegetables to ancient herbs and spices with aphrodisiac properties, you'll discover how to create enticing dishes that not only tantalize your taste buds but also contribute to your overall well-being.

The connection between diet and sexual health is not a new concept, but as we deepen our understanding of the intricate ways in which food influences our bodies, the significance of plant-based nutrition becomes increasingly evident. Join us on this culinary adventure as we unlock the secrets of plant-based diet cookbook offering you a roadmap to a healthier, more satisfying, and vibrant life. It's time to nourish not just your body but also your intimate well-being through the delectable wonders that nature provides.

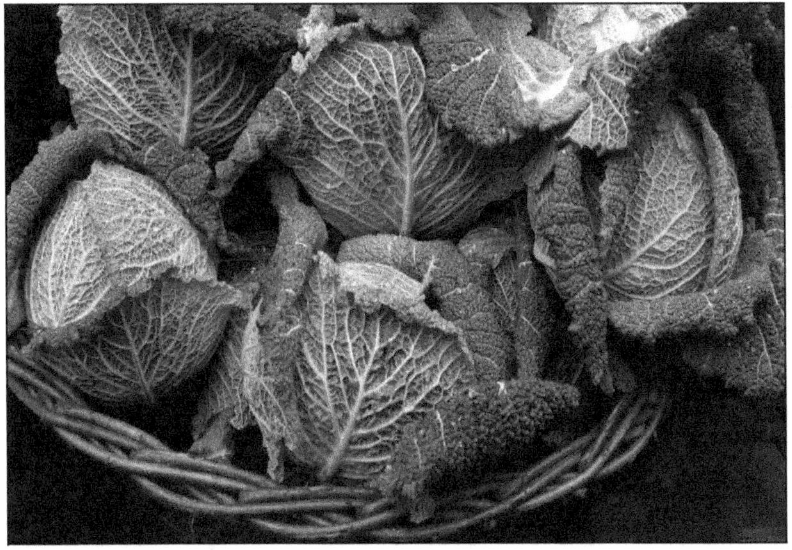

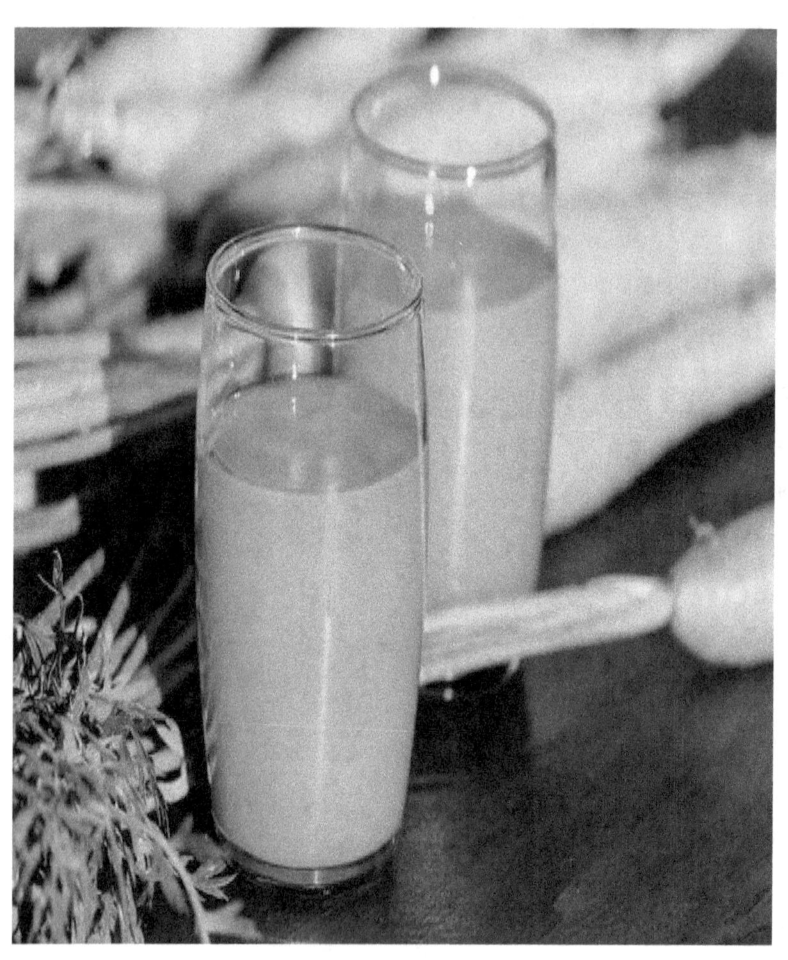

CHAPTER ONE

The Green Aphrodisiacs Unveiling the Power of Plants

The opening chapter of Plant-based Diet Cookbook for Seniors, we delve into the lush realm of green aphrodisiacs, where the vibrant colors of nature conceal a wealth of sexual wellness benefits. These verdant wonders not only tantalize the taste buds but also contribute to the enhancement of desire, performance, and overall vitality.

1.1 Leafy Greens

The Bedrock of Sexual Health

Explore the nutritional powerhouse found in leafy greens like spinach, kale, and Swiss chard. Packed with vitamins, minerals, and phytonutrients, these greens form the bedrock of sexual health by promoting a robust circulatory system, crucial for sustained arousal and performance.

1.2 Avocado

Nature's Creamy Elixir

Unlock the sensual potential of avocados, often referred to as nature's creamy elixir. Rich in monounsaturated fats and vitamin E, avocados contribute to improved cardiovascular health, supporting enhanced blood flow to vital regions and fostering a foundation for heightened intimacy.

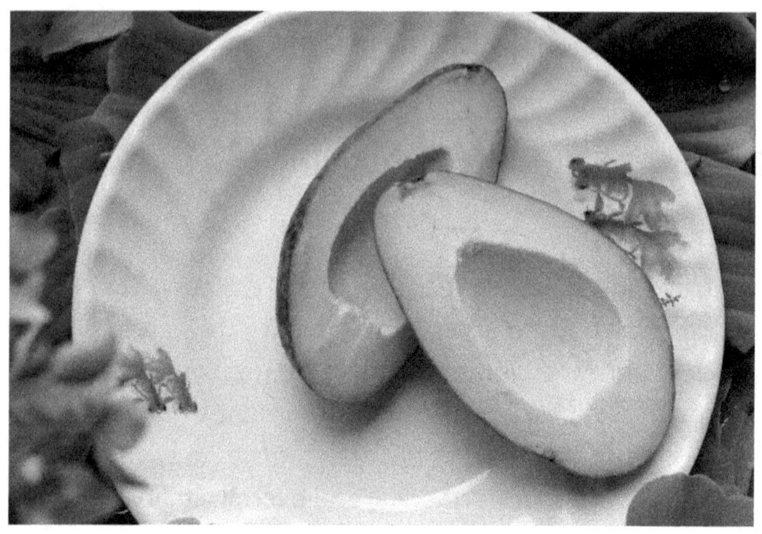

Creating vegan meals for seniors that focus on overall wellness, including sexual health, can be both delicious and nutritious. Here are a few recipes that align with the principles of the "Plant-Based Diet Cookbook for Seniors" and address low libido through wholesome, plant-based ingredients known to boost energy, circulation, and hormonal balance.

Avocado and Spinach Smoothie

Ingredients:

1 ripe avocado

2 cups fresh spinach

1 banana

1 cup almond milk (or any plant-based milk)

1 tablespoon chia seeds

1 teaspoon maca powder (known for boosting libido)Ice cubes (optional)

Instructions:

1.Cut the avocado in half, remove the pit, and scoop out the flesh.

2.In a blender, combine the avocado, spinach, banana, almond milk, chia seeds, and maca powder.

3.Blend until smooth. Add ice cubes if you prefer a chilled smoothie.

4.Serve immediately.

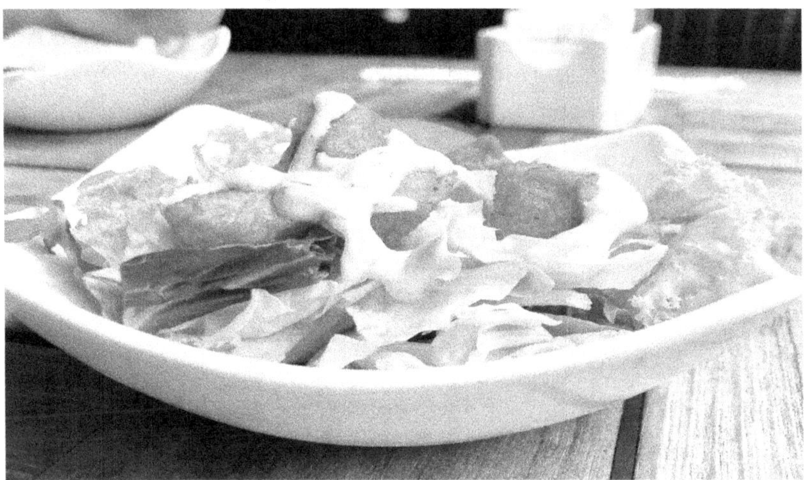

Quinoa and Roasted Vegetable Salad

Ingredients

1 cup quinoa, rinsed

2 cups water

1 red bell pepper, chopped

1 yellow bell pepper, chopped

1 zucchini, chopped

1 red onion, chopped

2 tablespoons olive oil

Salt and pepper to taste

1 cup cherry tomatoes, halved

1/4 cup fresh parsley, chopped

1/4 cup fresh basil, chopped

1 tablespoon balsamic vinegar

Instructions

1.Preheat the oven to 400°F (200°C).

2.Toss the bell peppers, zucchini, and red onion with olive oil, salt, and pepper. Spread on a baking sheet and roast for 20-25 minutes until tender.

3.Meanwhile, cook the quinoa by bringing the water to a boil. Add the quinoa, reduce heat, cover, and simmer for 15 minutes until water is absorbed. Fluff with a fork.

4.In a large bowl, combine the cooked quinoa, roasted vegetables, cherry tomatoes, parsley, and basil.

5.Drizzle with balsamic vinegar, toss, and serve.

Chickpea and Sweet Potato Curry

Ingredients

1 tablespoon coconut oil

1 onion, diced

3 garlic cloves, minced

1 tablespoon ginger, minced

1 tablespoon curry powder

1 teaspoon turmeric

1 teaspoon cumin

1 can (15 oz) chickpeas, drained and rinsed

2 medium sweet potatoes, peeled and cubed

1 can (14 oz) diced tomatoes
1 can (14 oz) coconut milk
Salt and pepper to taste

Fresh cilantro, chopped, for garnish
Instructions
1.In a large pot, heat the coconut oil over medium
heat. Add the onion, garlic, and ginger, and sauté until
the onion is translucent.
2.Stir in the curry powder, turmeric, and cumin,
cooking for another minute.
3.Add the chickpeas, sweet potatoes, diced tomatoes,
and coconut milk. Bring to a boil, then reduce heat
and simmer for 20-25 minutes until the sweet
potatoes are tender.
4.Season with salt and pepper to taste.
5.Serve hot, garnished with fresh cilantro.

Baked Tofu with Sesame and Ginger
Ingredients
1 block firm tofu, drained and pressed
2 tablespoons soy sauce or tamari
1 tablespoon sesame oil
1 tablespoon rice vinegar
1 tablespoon maple syrup
1 teaspoon grated ginger
1 teaspoon minced garlic
1 tablespoon sesame seeds
2 green onions, chopped

Instructions:

1. Preheat the oven to 375°F (190°C).
2. Cut the tofu into cubes and place in a single layer on a baking sheet lined with parchment paper.
3. In a small bowl, whisk together the soy sauce, sesame oil, rice vinegar, maple syrup, ginger, and garlic.
4. Pour the sauce over the tofu cubes, ensuring they are well coated. Sprinkle with sesame seeds.
5. Bake for 25-30 minutes until the tofu is golden and slightly crispy.
6. Garnish with chopped green onions before serving.

Berry Chia Pudding

Ingredients

1/4 cup chia seeds

1 cup almond milk (or any plant-based milk)

1 tablespoon maple syrup

1/2 teaspoon vanilla extract

1 cup mixed berries {blueberries, strawberries, raspberries}

Fresh mint leaves for garnish (optional)

Instructions

1. In a bowl, mix the chia seeds, almond milk, maple syrup, and vanilla extract. Stir well to combine.
2. Cover and refrigerate for at least 4 hours, or overnight, until the mixture thickens to a pudding-like consistency.
3. Stir the pudding to break up any clumps. Serve topped with mixed berries and garnish with fresh mint leaves if desired. These recipes provide a variety of

nutrients that can help improve overall health and well-being for seniors, including enhancing sexual wellness. Enjoy!

1.1 Asparagus Stalks of Desire

Delve into the symbolism and substance of asparagus, celebrated through the ages as a symbol of desire. Discover how this slender, green vegetable is not just a culinary delight but also a source of folate and potassium, essential for maintaining reproductive health and hormone balance.

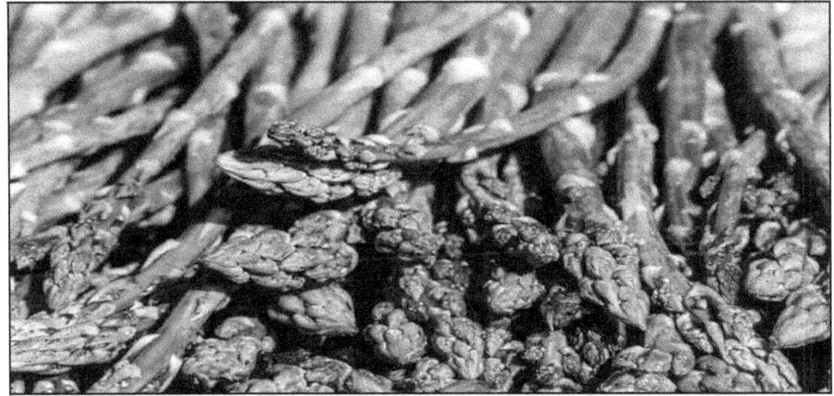

Explore the cruciferous wonders such as broccoli, cauliflower, and Brussels sprouts, known for their hormone-balancing properties. These vegetables contain compounds that support the liver's detoxification processes, playing a pivotal role in hormonal harmony and contributing to overall sexual wellness.

1.2 Spirulina and Algae The Oceanic Potency

Venture into the aquatic realm with spirulina and algae, harnessing the power of these plant-like organisms rich in amino acids, vitamins, and minerals. Discover how incorporating these green treasures into your diet can provide essential nutrients that may boost energy levels and promote sustained stamina.As we navigate the verdant landscapes of these green aphrodisiacs, we uncover not only their culinary versatility but also their potential to fortify the foundations of sexual vitality. Join us in this exploration of nature's green bounty, where the key to unlocking a plant-based diet cookbook lies within the vibrant spectrum of nutrient-dense, delicious greens.

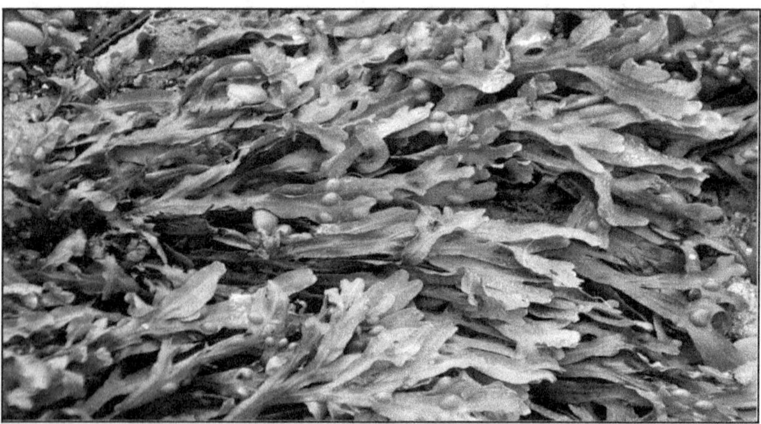

Sowing the Seeds of Vigor: Nuts, Seeds, And Your Sexual Health

Embark on a journey into the world of nuts and seeds, where we unveil their potential to sow the seeds of vigor in your sexual health. Packed with essential fatty acids, vitamins, and minerals, these small yet mighty ingredients play a crucial role in supporting reproductive function, promoting stamina, and boosting overall energy. Discover the art of incorporating chia seeds, pumpkin seeds, and almonds into your daily diet to cultivate robust sexual well-being. The Plant-based diet cookbook for seniors we embark on a journey into the world of nuts and seeds, exploring how these miniature marvels hold the key to sowing the seeds of vigor in your sexual health. Bursting with essential nutrients, healthy fats, and a symphony of flavors, nuts and seeds become the protagonists in your quest for enhanced vitality and enduring sexual wellness.

2.1 Chia Seeds Tiny Powerhouses of Nutrient Density

Discover the potential of chia seeds, tiny yet mighty powerhouses known for their exceptional nutrient density. Rich in omega-3 fatty acids, fiber, and protein, chia seeds contribute to cardiovascular health, promoting robust blood circulation—an essential factor in achieving and sustaining arousal.

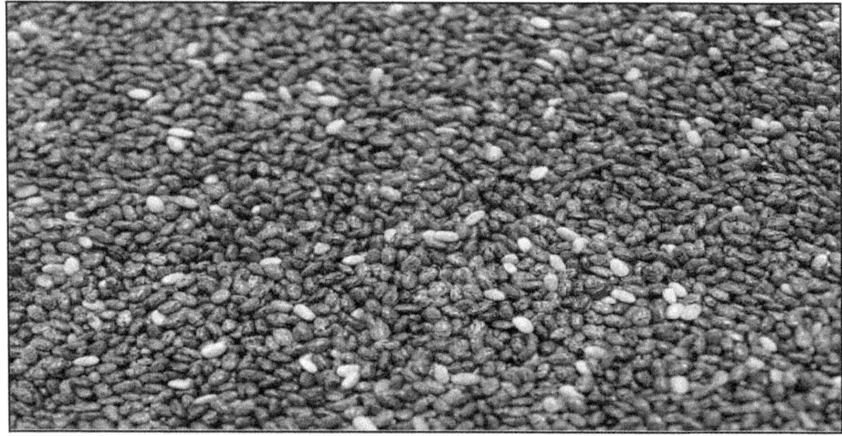

2.2 Pumpkin Seeds A Zinc-Rich Elixir for Male Vitality

Delve into the masculine virtues of pumpkin seeds, celebrated for their abundance of zinc—an essential mineral crucial for testosterone production. Discover how incorporating these seeds into your diet may play a pivotal role in maintaining hormonal balance, supporting reproductive health, and fostering overall male vitality.

2.3 Almonds Nutrient-Rich Ambrosia for Endurance

Explore the world of almonds, a nutrient-rich ambrosia renowned for its versatility and sexual wellness benefits. Packed with vitamin E, magnesium, and antioxidants, almonds contribute to improved blood flow, stamina, and overall endurance—making them an invaluable addition to your daily dietary repertoire.

2.4 Flaxseeds: Omega-3 Rich Allies for Hormonal Harmony

Unlock the potential of flaxseeds, omega-3 rich allies that promote hormonal harmony within the body. Delve into their role in supporting a healthy balance of estrogen and testosterone, contributing to reproductive health and potentially enhancing libido.

2.5 Sesame Seeds Tiny Troves of Nutrient Goodness

Embark on a culinary adventure with sesame seeds, tiny troves of nutrient goodness packed with zinc, magnesium, and iron. Discover how these unassuming seeds can add a delightful crunch to your dishes while nurturing your body with essential minerals that play a role in sexual health. As we explore the myriad benefits of nuts and seeds, this will unveil the potential of these wholesome additions to foster vigor and vitality in your sexual journey. From chia's nutrient density to pumpkin seeds' zinc-rich elixir, each seed contributes its unique essence to the symphony of plant-based diet cookbook. Welcome to a chapter where the humble seeds become the catalysts for sowing the seeds of vigor in your pursuit of enduring sexual wellness.

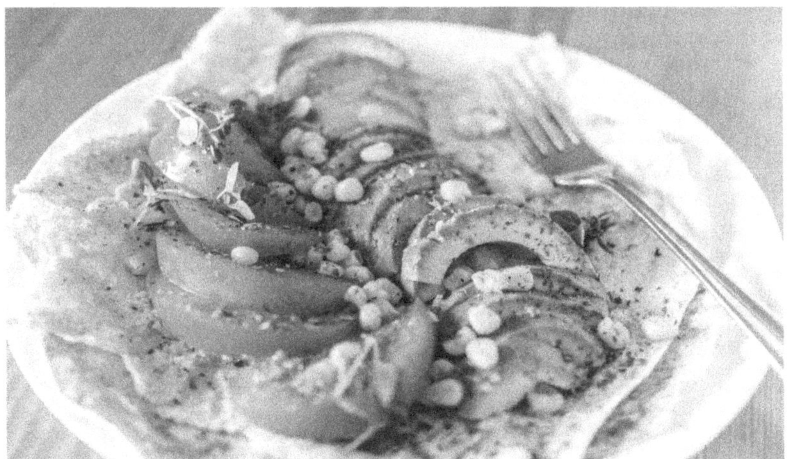

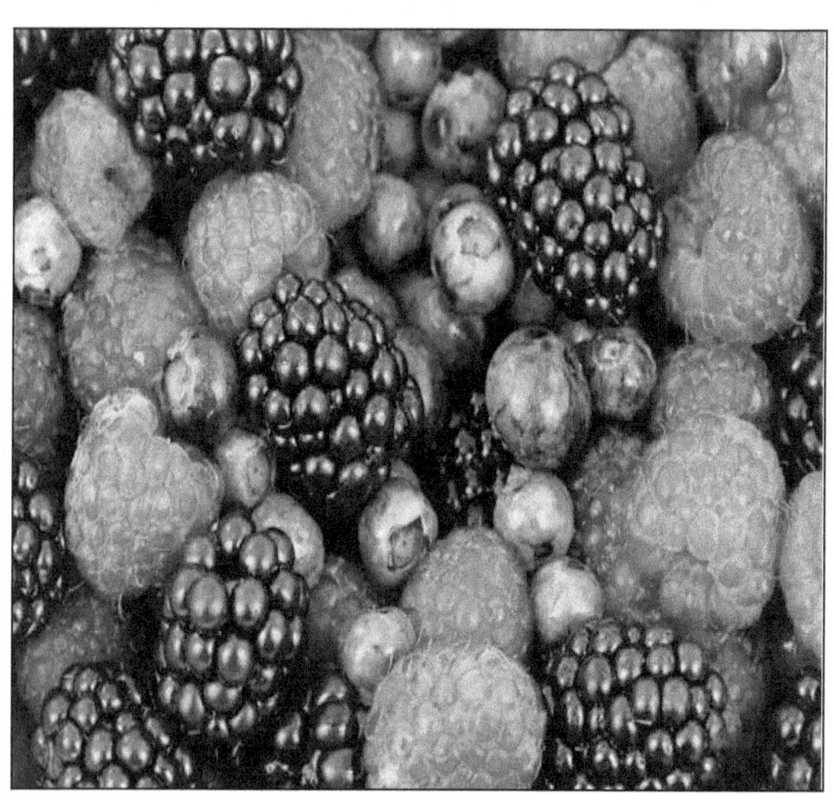

CHAPTER TWO

Fruits of Passion Sweet Sensations for Sensual Satisfaction

Delve into the sweet and succulent world of fruits that not only tantalize your taste buds but also heighten your sensual satisfaction. From the antioxidant-rich berries to the potassium-packed bananas and the juicy watermelon, learn how these fruits contribute to improved blood flow, arousal, and endurance. Uncover delightful recipes that seamlessly integrate these fruits into your meals, turning each bite into a celebration of pleasure and vitality. In the enchanting landscape of The Plant-based diet cookbook our culinary exploration continues with the irresistible allure of fruits—nature's sweet sensations that not only captivate your taste buds but also contribute to sensual satisfaction. From succulent berries to exotic tropical delights, this chapter unveils the diverse array of fruits that play a vital role in enhancing desire, improving circulation, and fostering an environment of blissful intimacy.

3.1 Berries Antioxidant-rich Jewels of Desire

Embark on a journey through the world of berries—blueberries, strawberries, raspberries, and more—celebrated not only for their vibrant flavors but also for their high levels of antioxidants. Discover how these jewel-like fruits contribute to improved blood flow, reducing oxidative stress and providing a foundation for heightened desire.

Nature's Phallic Elixir 3.2 Bananas

Uncover the symbolism and substance of bananas, nature's phallic elixir. Rich in potassium, vitamins, and natural sugars, bananas contribute to sustained energy levels and support cardiovascular health, factors essential for endurance and maintaining arousal.

3.3 Watermelon: Juicy Hydration and Libido Boost

Dive into the juicy world of watermelon, a hydrating delight that holds a surprising secret. Learn how this summertime favorite, with its high-water content and citrulline content, may contribute to improved blood flow, potentially enhancing libido and creating a refreshing addition to your sensual repertoire.

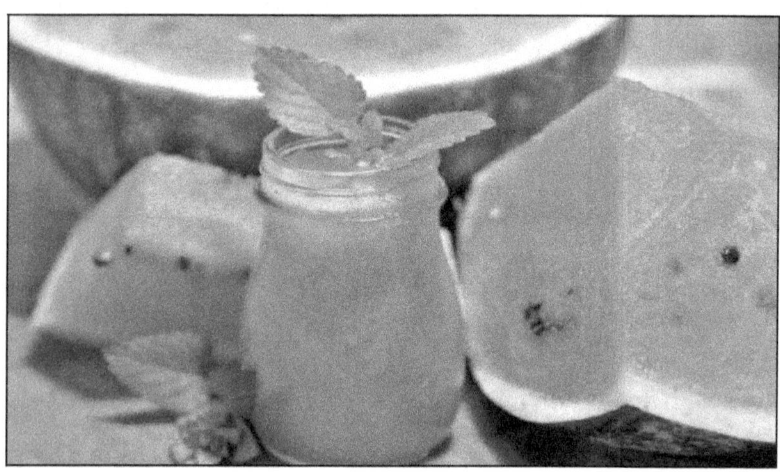

3.4 Mangoes: Exotic Treasures of Passion

Indulge in the exotic allure of mangoes, not just as a tropical delight but as a source of vitamins A and E, known for their potential to enhance skin health and contribute to a sensuous touch. Discover how this luscious fruit can add a touch of passion to your culinary creations.

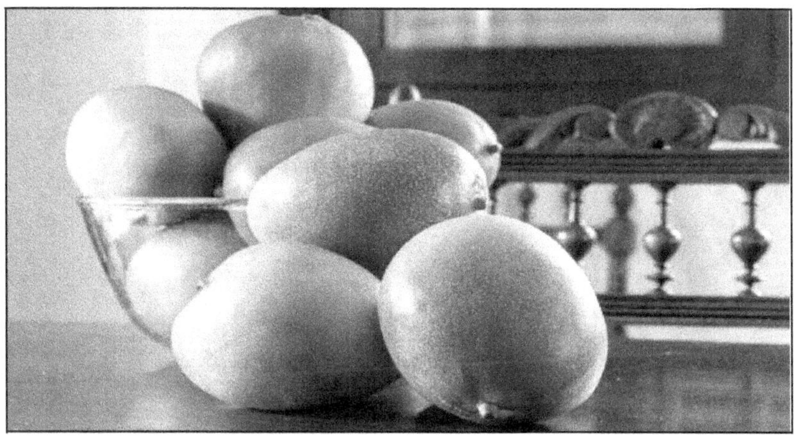

Explore the jewel-toned allure of pomegranates, revered as aphrodisiacs for centuries. Delve into their rich antioxidant content, which may support cardiovascular health, improve blood flow, and add a burst of passion to your intimate moments.

As we immerse ourselves in the sweet sensations of fruits, this chapter invites you to savor the delectable symphony of flavors while unlocking the potential for enhanced desire and sensual satisfaction. From the antioxidant-rich berries to the juicy allure of watermelon, each fruit becomes a delightful addition to your journey toward a plant-based diet cookbook and a more fulfilling intimate life. Welcome to a chapter where the fruits of passion become not just a feast for the senses but also allies in your pursuit of heightened sexual wellness.

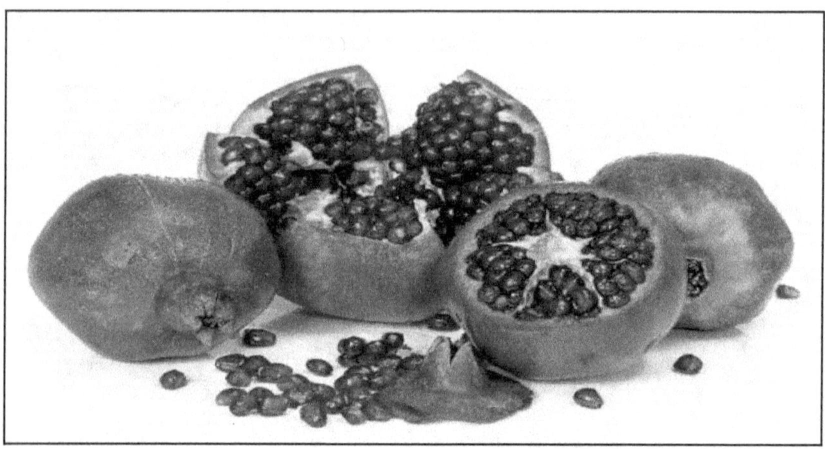

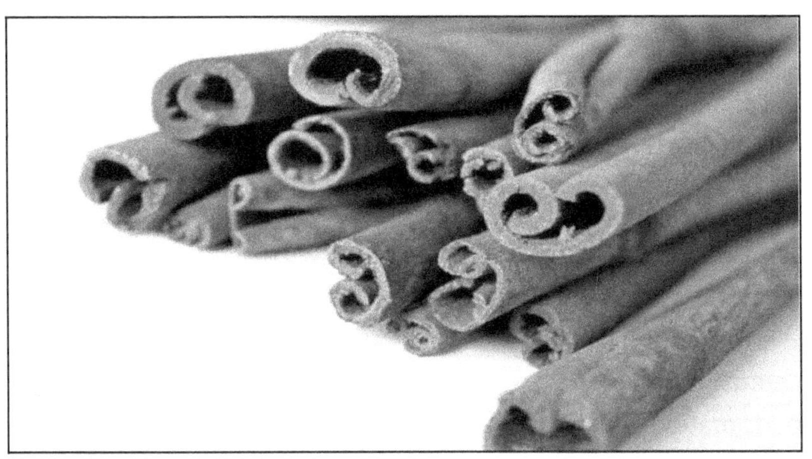

Spice Up Your Love Life Culinary Adventures with Aphrodisiac Herbs and Spices

Embark on a culinary adventure with a diverse range of aphrodisiac herbs and spices that have been celebrated for centuries for their role in enhancing desire and intimacy. From the exotic saffron to the warming effects of cinnamon, discover how these flavorful additions can not only elevate the taste of your dishes but also spice up your love life by promoting circulation, balancing hormones, and sparking passion. In the aromatic realm of Plant-based diet cookbook for seniors, our culinary exploration takes a captivating turn as we delve into the world of aphrodisiac herbs and spices. Discover how these flavorful treasures not only elevate the taste of your dishes but also spark passion, stimulate circulation, and contribute to a heightened sense of intimacy. Get ready to embark on a culinary adventure that transforms your kitchen into a haven of love and desire.

The Golden Elixir of Love

Embark on a journey with saffron, the golden elixir that has adorned love stories throughout history. Explore the delicate threads of this prized spice, known for its exotic aroma and potential mood-enhancing properties. Uncover how saffron may contribute to relaxation and the creation of an intimate atmosphere.

Cinnamon

Aromatic Spice of Warmth and Desire

Savor the warmth and desire infused by cinnamon as we navigate its aromatic allure. Discover how this spice, with its rich history and versatile flavor profile, can not only add depth to your culinary creations but also potentially stimulate blood flow and heighten sensations.

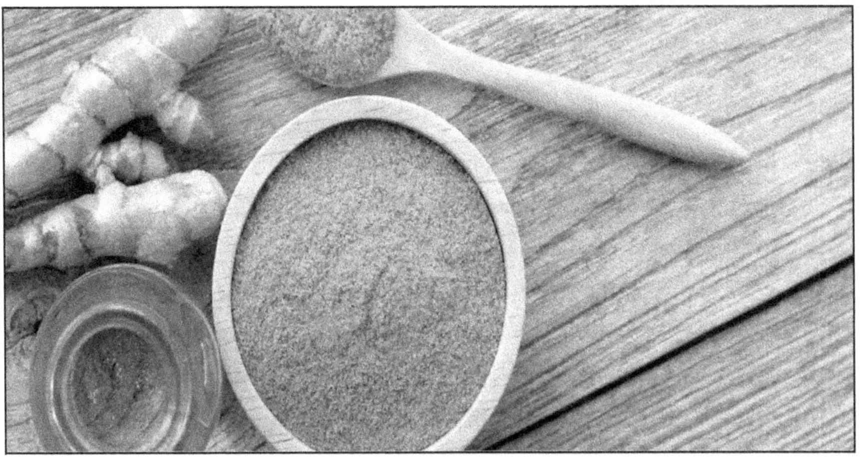

CHAPTER THREE

Ginger The Zing of Passionate Heat

Feel the zing of passionate heat with ginger, a spice celebrated for its bold flavor and potential health benefits. From its warming properties to its anti-inflammatory effects, ginger adds a fiery element to both your cuisine and your intimate moments, stimulating the senses in more ways than one.

Cardamom Fragrant Pods of Sensuality

Uncover the fragrant pods of cardamom, celebrated for their aromatic richness and potential aphrodisiac qualities. Explore how this spice, with its unique blend of sweet and spicy notes, can add a layer of sensuality to your dishes while potentially contributing to improved digestion—a key factor in overall well-being.

Vanilla Sweet Euphoria in Every Pod

Delve into the sweet euphoria of vanilla, a timeless and indulgent spice that transcends its culinary role. Discover how vanilla, with its comforting aroma, may create a sense of intimacy and relaxation, transforming your meals into delightful experiences for the senses. As we navigate the rich tapestry of aphrodisiac herbs and spices, this chapter invites you to infuse your culinary creations with passion and desire. From the golden threads of saffron to the sweet euphoria of vanilla, each spice becomes a culinary ally in your pursuit of a plant-based diet cookbook and a more enchanting love life. Welcome to a chapter where the aromatic wonders of the kitchen become the catalysts for spicing up your love life.

Crafting Elixirs of Love: Plant-Powered Beverages for Blissful Nights

Plant-based diet cookbook for seniors, we immerse ourselves in the art of crafting elixirs that go beyond mere refreshment, offering you plant-powered beverages designed to enhance your intimate moments. From soothing herbal teas to nutrient-packed smoothies, join us in exploring concoctions that not only nourish your body but also contribute to a blissful night of pleasure and connection.

Hibiscus and Rose Infusion

A Floral Symphony for Romance

Embark on a journey into the world of floral infusions with hibiscus and rose. Discover how the vibrant hues and delicate aromas of these flowers create a symphony that not only pleases the senses but also potentially contributes to improved circulation and relaxation, setting the stage

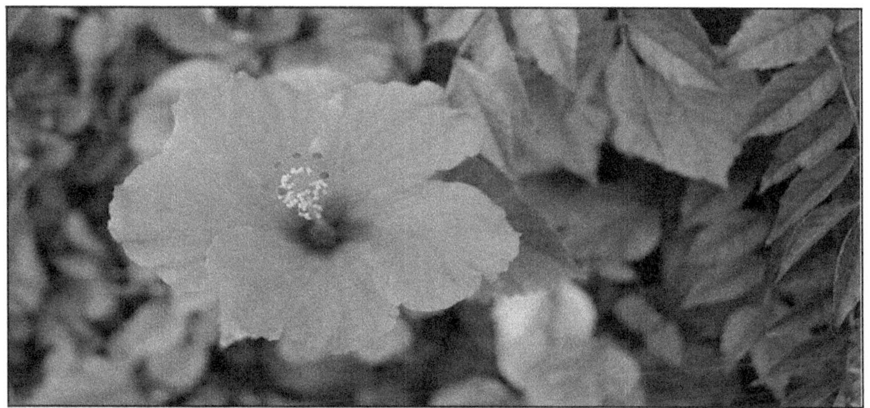

for an intimate evening.

Maca and Cacao Smoothie Energizing Elixirs for Passionate Nights

Savor the rich flavors of maca and cacao in a delectable smoothie that not only tantalizes your taste buds but also energizes your body. Discover the potential benefits of maca root for stamina and hormonal balance, while the indulgence of cacao adds a touch of decadence to your romantic rendezvous.

Turmeric Golden Milk Anti-Inflammatory Elixir for Tranquil Evenings

Delve into the comforting warmth of turmeric golden milk, a soothing elixir celebrated for its anti-inflammatory properties. Explore how the combination of turmeric, ginger, and other spices can create a beverage that not only promotes relaxation but also supports overall well-being, creating a tranquil ambiance for shared moments.

Pineapple and Mint Sparkler Refreshing Libations for Intimate Celebrations

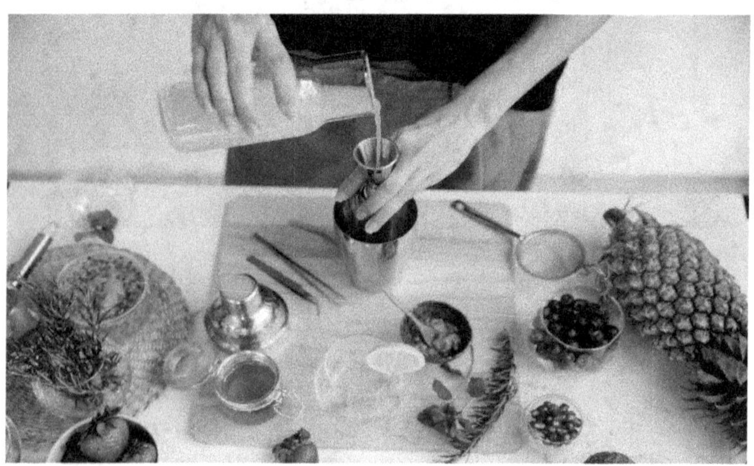

Celebrate the refreshing combination of pineapple and mint in a sparkling elixir that invigorates your senses. Discover how the enzymes in pineapple may contribute to digestion, while the invigorating essence of mint adds a crisp touch to your intimate celebrations,leaving you refreshed and rejuvenated.

Green Tea Elixirs

Antioxidant-rich Brews for Sipping Pleasure

Explore the world of green tea elixirs, where antioxidants and subtle flavors combine to create beverages that not only provide a moment of respite but also contribute to cardiovascular health. Uncover the potential benefits of green tea in promoting relaxation and enhancing the mood for shared moments of pleasure. As we progress our journey through this chapter and invite you to raise a glass to the culmination of flavors, aromas, and potential benefits that plant-powered beverages can bring to your intimate life. From floral infusions to energizing smoothies, each elixir becomes a delightful companion in your pursuit of a blissful night of passion and connection. Welcome to a chapter where the craft of elixirs of love becomes a celebration of plant powered pleasure

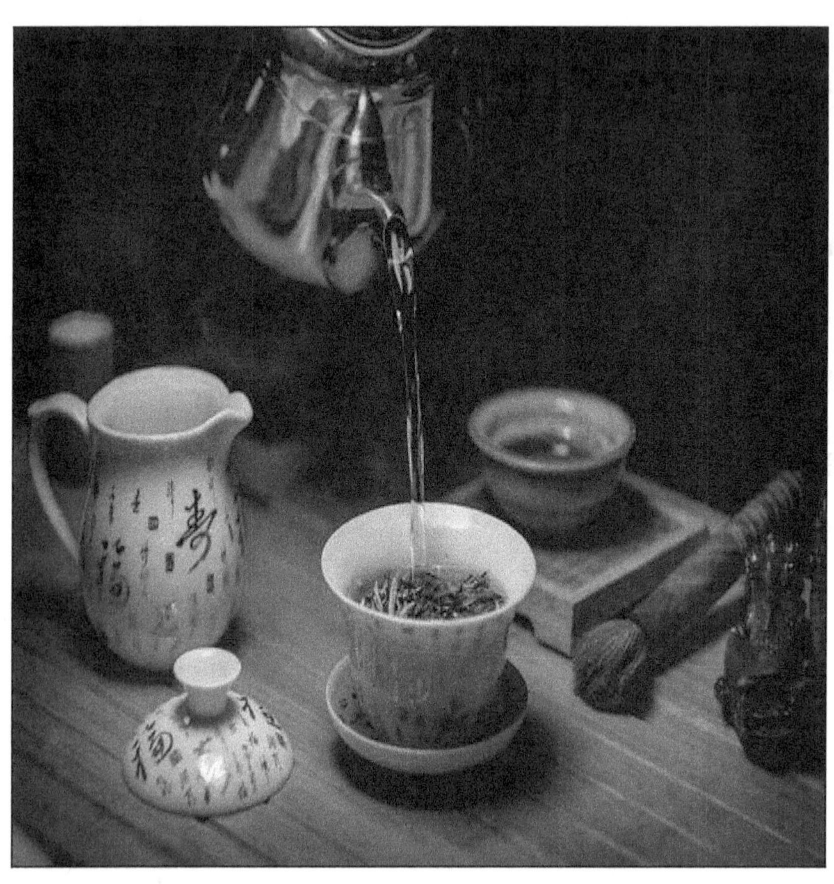

CHAPTER FOUR

The Energy Elixirs

Welcome to the heart of plant-powered vitality! In this section, we unlock the secrets to boosting your energy and invigorating your sexual wellness through a tantalizing array of Energy Elixirs. These carefully curated recipes are crafted with a blend of nature's most potent ingredients to elevate your stamina and performance.

1. Morning Mojo Smoothie

Kickstart your day with a delicious concoction of maca root, banana, spinach, and almond milk. This powerhouse smoothie is packed with libido-boosting nutrients and antioxidants, providing sustained energy to fuel your daily activities and amorous adventures.

2. Ginseng Infusion

Harness the ancient power of ginseng in this revitalizing tea. Known for its adaptogen properties, ginseng helps combat stress and fatigue while enhancing overall vitality. Sip on this elixir throughout the day to maintain a steady flow of energy and mental clarity.

3. Passion Fruit Power Shot

A concentrated burst of passion fruit, ginger, and turmeric creates a potent elixir to fuel your passion. The anti-inflammatory properties of turmeric combined with the invigorating kick of ginger make this shot a must-have in your arsenal for enhanced endurance.

4. Cacao Libido Latte

Indulge in the decadent richness of cacao, blended with warming spices and a touch of plant-based milk. Cacao is renowned for its ability to stimulate the release of endorphins, promoting a positive mood and enhancing the pleasure of intimate moments.

5. Pomegranate Punch

Revel in the sweet and tart goodness of pomegranate paired with a hint of mint. Pomegranates are celebrated for their potential to improve blood circulation, contributing to increased vitality and endurance. Each recipe in this section is designed not only to tantalize your taste buds but also to infuse your body with the natural energy it needs. As you incorporate these Energy Elixirs into your routine, you'll find yourself not just energized but ready to embrace the full spectrum of your sexual well-being. and a fulfilling life!

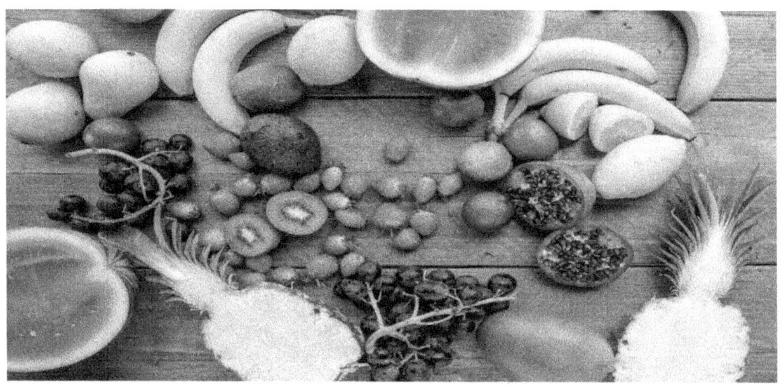

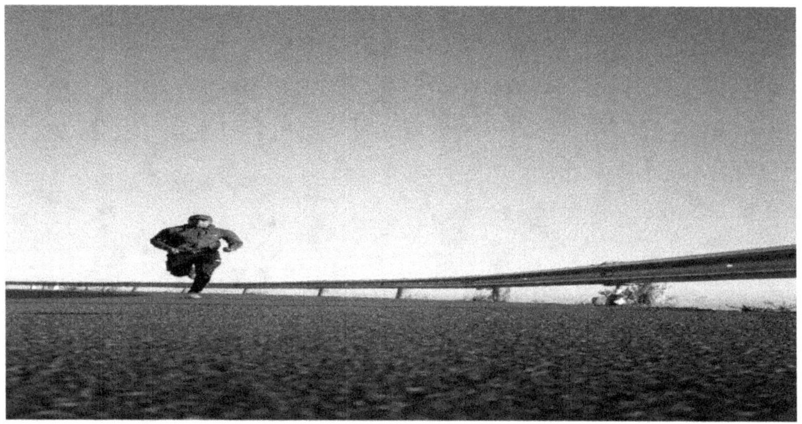

Nutrient-Rich Breakfasts for Libido

Start your day right with nutrient-dense breakfast options that not only satisfy your taste buds but also fuel your body for optimal sexual wellness. Explore creative and delicious plant-based recipes featuring ingredients known for their aphrodisiac properties. These meals are designed to provide sustained energy and promote overall sexual health. Rise and shine with a breakfast that not only satisfies your taste buds but also fuels the fire of your desire! This section is dedicated to exploring nutrient-rich breakfast options designed to kickstart your day and enhance your libido. Packed with wholesome ingredients, these recipes are a delicious invitation to prioritize your sexual wellness from the very beginning.

Quinoa Power Porridge

Begin your day with a protein-packed bowl of quinoa, adorned with fresh berries, nuts, and a drizzle of honey. This hearty porridge not only provides essential nutrients but also supports sustained energy throughout the day, promoting a healthy libido.

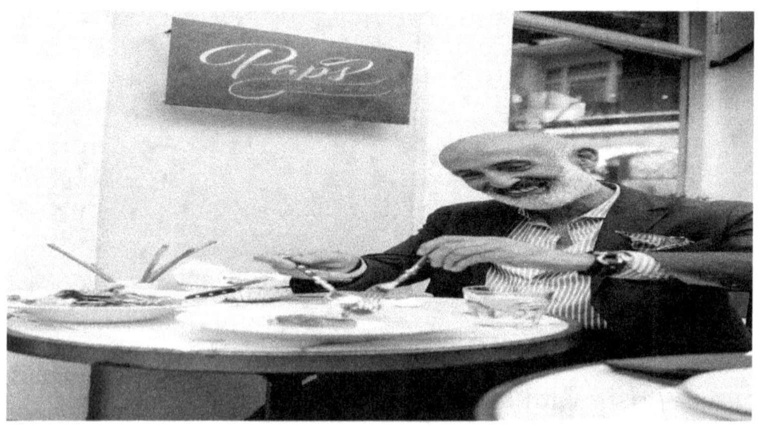

Avocado & Tomato Toast Delight

Elevate your classic avocado toast by adding juicy tomatoes and a sprinkle of pumpkin seeds. Avocados are rich in monounsaturated fats, which contribute to improved blood flow—a key factor in maintaining sexual health.

Chia Seed Pudding Parfait

Dive into layers of chia seed pudding, Greek yogurt, and a medley of tropical fruits. Chia seeds are a nutritional powerhouse, offering omega-3 fatty acids and fiber, which contribute to heart health and overall vitality—essential for a thriving libido

Sweet Potato and Spinach Frittata

Unleash the power of vitamin-rich sweet potatoes and iron-packed spinach in a delicious frittata. These ingredients support healthy blood circulation and are known to enhance stamina, laying the foundation for a satisfying and energetic day.

Banana Walnut Pancakes

Savor the sweetness of banana and the crunch of walnuts in a stack of wholesome pancakes. Bananas are rich in potassium, which helps regulate blood pressure, fostering cardiovascular health and, in turn, supporting optimal sexual function.

By incorporating these nutrient-rich breakfasts into your routine, you're not just nourishing your body but also nurturing your libido. The journey to enhanced sexual

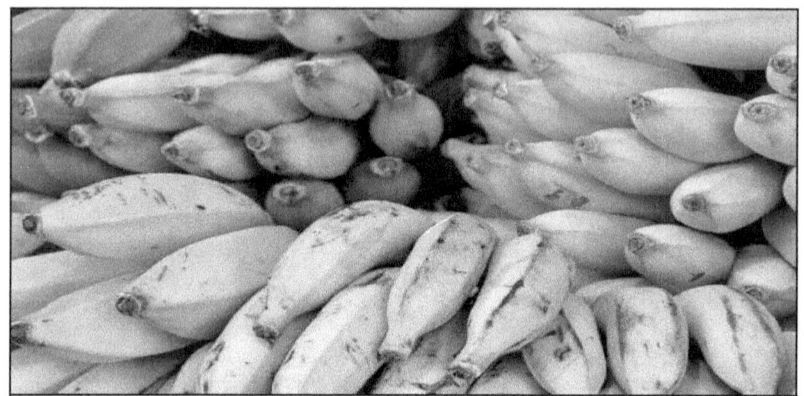

wellness begins with the first meal of the day, setting a positive tone for the experiences that follow. Enjoy the pleasure of these breakfast creations and embrace a lifestyle that prioritizes both your palate and your passion.

CHAPTER FIVE

Superfoods and Sensuality

Uncover the role of superfoods in enhancing sensuality. This page delves into the nutritional benefits of specific plant-based superfoods that have been traditionally linked to improved sexual function. Learn how incorporating these ingredients into your diet can contribute to increased libido, better circulation, and overall reproductive health

Embark on a journey through the realm of superfoods, where nutritional power meets sensuality. This section delves into the extraordinary benefits of specific plant-based superfoods, each carefully chosen for its ability to amplify sensuality and contribute to overall sexual well-being. Discover how these extraordinary ingredients can elevate your intimate experiences to new heights.

Acai Berry Bliss Bowl

Immerse yourself in the antioxidant-rich goodness of acai berries, topped with nuts, seeds, and a drizzle of honey. Acai berries not only combat oxidative stress but also promote healthy blood flow—an essential factor in enhancing sensuality.

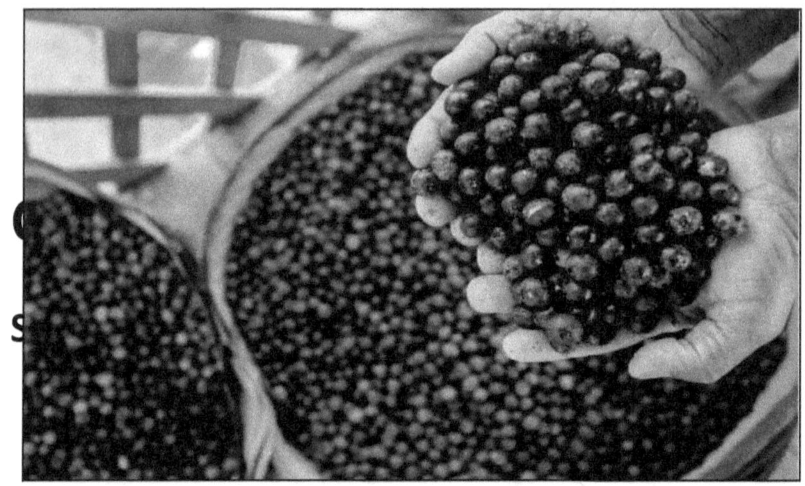

Experience the vibrant green energy of spirulina blended into a refreshing smoothie with pineapple, mango, and coconut water. Spirulina's nutrient density provides a boost of essential vitamins and minerals, supporting both physical and mental well-being.

Passion Bites

Indulge in decadent bites infused with the energy-boosting power of maca root. **Maca** is celebrated for its ability to enhance stamina and libido, making it a perfect addition to your arsenal of superfoods for sensuality.

Goji Berry Elixir

Sip on a tantalizing elixir made with goji berries, citrus, and a hint of mint. Goji berries are known for their antioxidant properties and potential benefits in promoting sexual

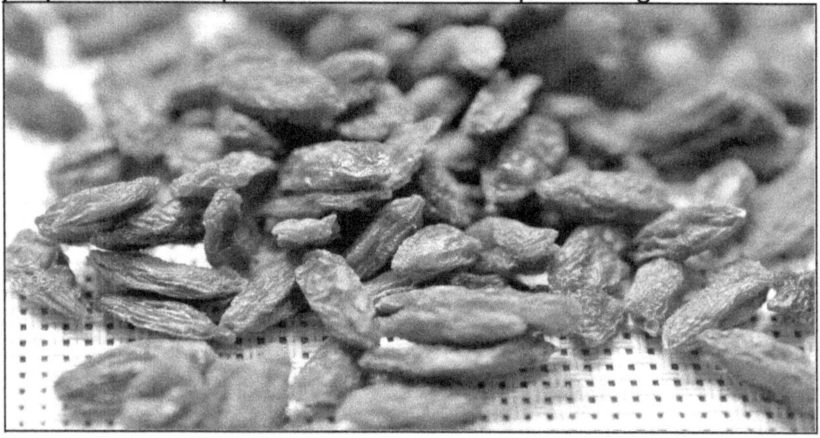

Turmeric Infused Love Latte

Delight in the warming embrace of turmeric, ginger, and a touch of cinnamon in a velvety latte. Turmeric's anti-inflammatory properties may contribute to increased blood flow, promoting a heightened sense of pleasure. As you explore the world of superfoods and sensuality, remember that the path to enhanced intimacy is paved with the mindful incorporation of these nutrient-packed delights. Elevate your culinary experiences and embrace the extraordinary benefits that nature's superfoods bring to your overall well-being and sensuality.

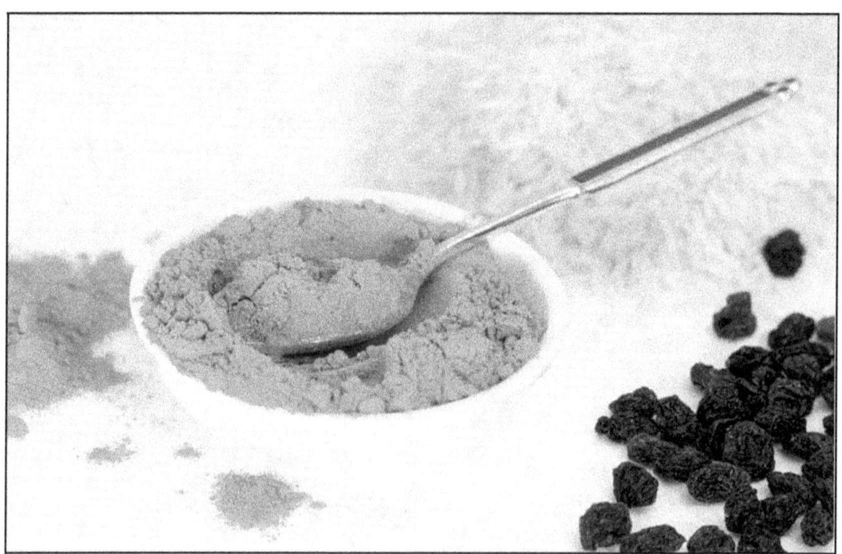

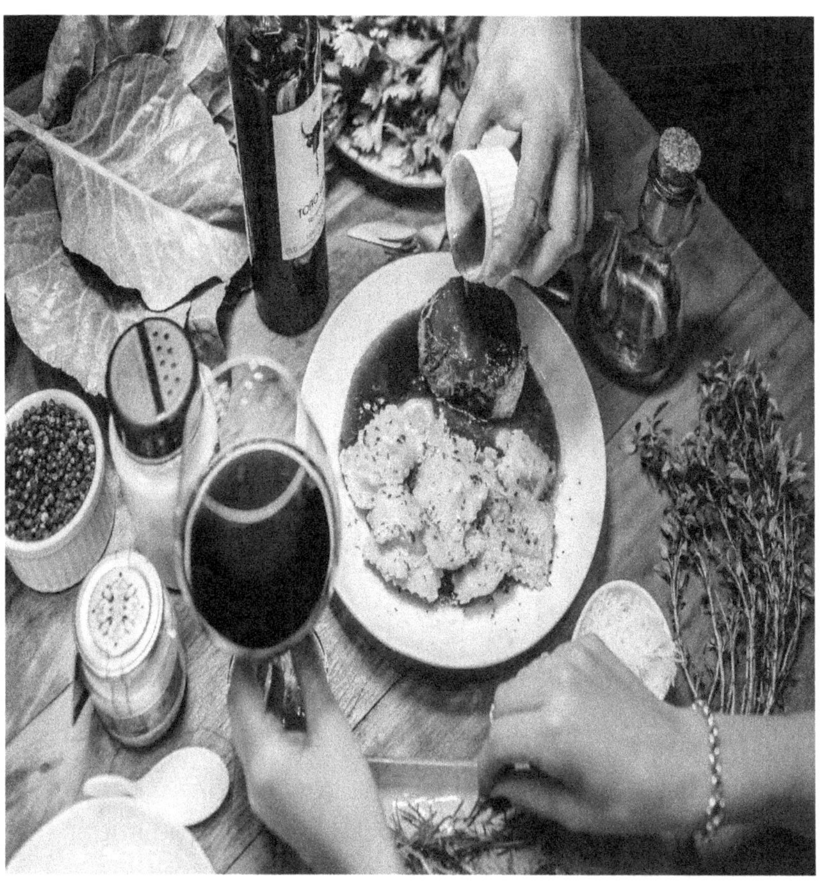

Mindful Eating

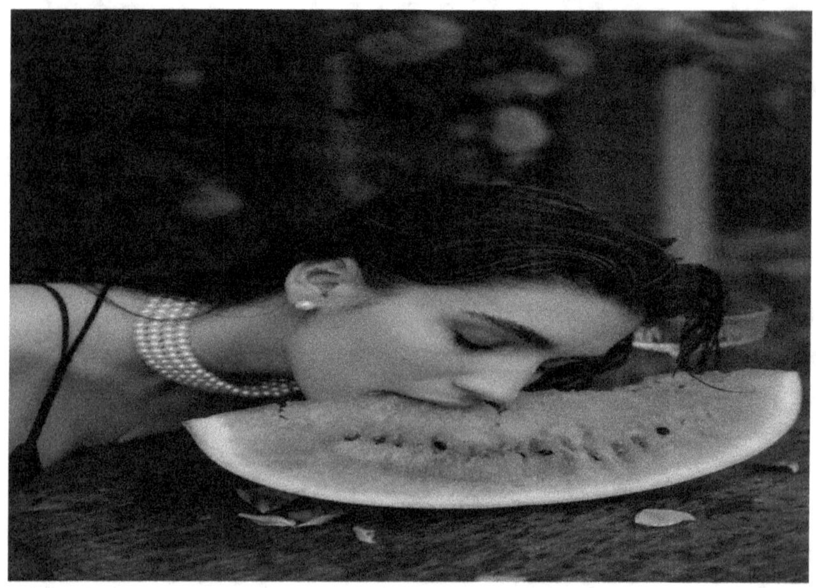

Eating fresh watermelon and seeds too offers their own holistic health benefits. it helps slow down sugar absorption in the gut and mellows the rise in blood sugar and boost athletic performance. Beyond the physical aspects, this section explores the connection between mindful eating and heightened intimacy. Understand the importance of being present in the moment and savoring each bite. Learn techniques to cultivate mindfulness, promoting a deeper connection with both your food and your partner. Discover how conscious eating can positively impact your sexual well-being. As you progress through these pages, the cookbook aims to empower men with a holistic approach to sexual wellness, emphasizing the significance of nourishing the body with plant-based ingredients for a healthier and more satisfying intimate life.

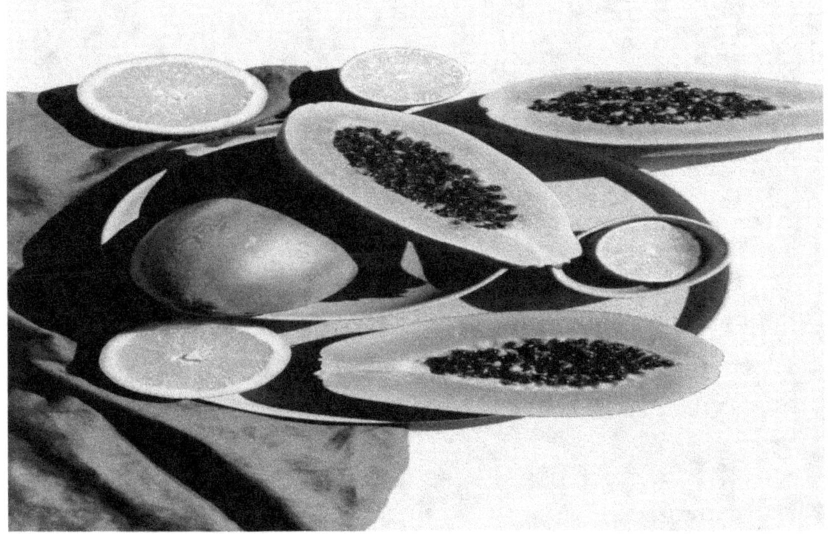

Welcome to the transformative practice of mindful eating, a key to unlocking deeper connections both with your food and your partner. In this section, we explore the profound impact that conscious consumption can have on your intimate experiences. Discover the art of savoring each bite, cultivating presence, and fostering a deeper connection with yourself and your loved one.

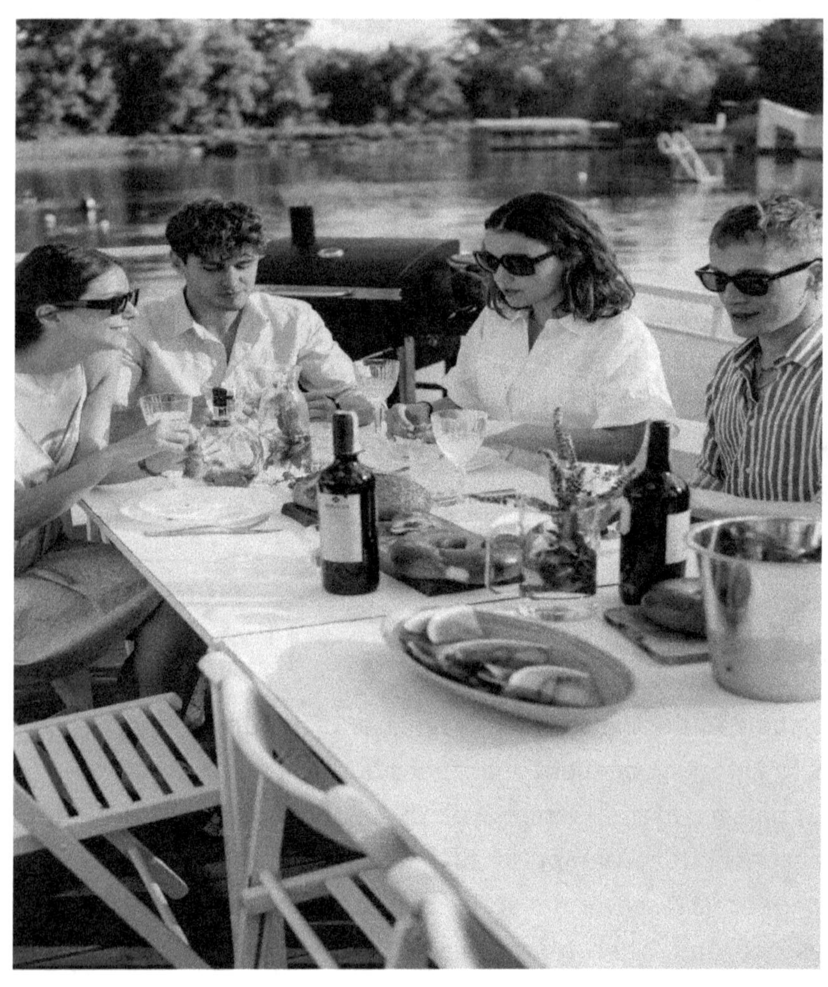

CHAPTER SIX

The Ritual of Preparation

Begin your journey into mindful eating by appreciating the art of food preparation. Engage your senses as you chop, mix, and create, turning meal preparation into a meditative experience. This intentional approach sets the stage for a mindful and pleasurable dining experience.

Present Moment Awareness

Explore the concept of being fully present at the table. Banish distractions, put away electronic devices, and focus on the sensory experience of eating. Engage with the textures, flavors, and aromas of your food, allowing each moment to unfold without the interference of external distractions.

Gratitude and Nourishment

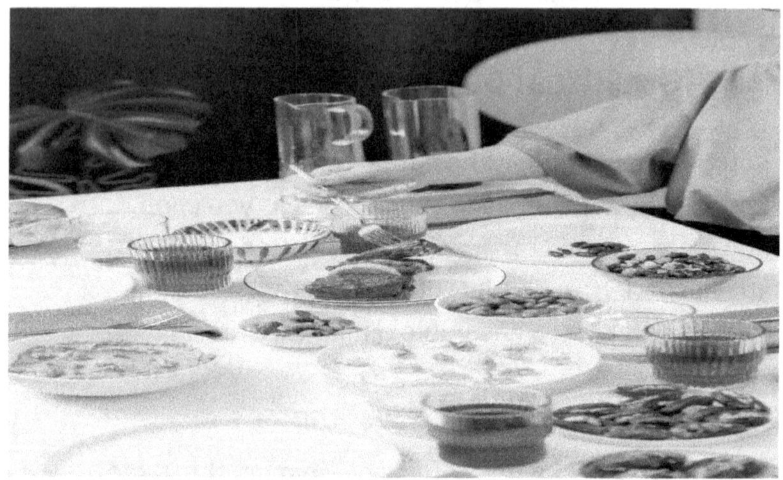

Cultivate gratitude for the nourishment that each meal provides. Reflect on the journey of the ingredients from farm to table, acknowledging the effort and energy that went into bringing sustenance to your plate. Expressing gratitude can elevate the act of eating to a sacred and fulfilling experience. Certainly, a book on plant-based potency for men aged 40-65. Keep in mind that the actual content and organization would depend on the specific goals and approach of the book. Here's a suggested outline:

Nutritional Support for Seniors Sexual Health.

Discussing the role of nutrition in overall health and its specific impact on sexual wellness.

Emphasizes on the importance of a balanced and plant-based diet.

Key Nutrients for Men's Sexual Health

Explore nutrients crucial for male sexual function, such as zinc, vitamin D, omega-3 fatty acids, and antioxidants. Provide information on plant-based sources of these nutrients.

Adapting the Diet for Aging Men

Address the changing nutritional needs as men age. discuss strategies for incorporating nutrient-dense plant-based foods into the diet. Herbs and Supplements. Explore plant-based supplements and herbs known for their potential benefits in supporting sexual health. Highlight scientific studies supporting the effectiveness of these supplements.

Lifestyle Factors and Sexual Wellness

Exercise and Physical Activity

Discuss the role of regular exercise in maintaining sexual health. Provide examples of plant-based protein sources for muscle health.

Stress Management

Explore the connection between chronic stress and sexual dysfunction. Introduce mindfulness techniques and stress-reducing practices.

Sleep and Sexual Health

Highlight the importance of adequate sleep for hormonal balance and overall well-being. Provide tips for improving sleep quality.

Limiting Unhealthy Habits

Discuss the negative impact of smoking, excessive alcohol consumption, and   other unhealthy habits on sexual function. Provide guidance on reducing or eliminating these behaviors.

Mind-Body Connection

Explore the interconnectedness of mental and physical health in relation to sexual wellness.

Introduce practices like meditation and yoga.

Communication and Relationships

Discuss the importance of open communication with partners about sexual health. Address relationship dynamics and their impact on sexual well-being.

Medical Considerations and Consultation

Encourage regular check-ups and screenings for potential health issues. Emphasize the importance of consulting healthcare professionals for personalized advice.

Future Directions and Emerging Research

Highlight ongoing research in plant-based solutions for men's sexual health. Discuss potential future developments in the field. Remember, the above is a general outline, and the actual content would require detailed research and customization based on the book's specific goals and audience.

Sharing and Connection

Embrace the communal aspect of dining. Share your thoughts, feelings, and experiences with your partner as you enjoy the meal together. Communication and connection during meals foster a sense of intimacy, allowing you to strengthen your bond through shared moments of pleasure.

Sensory Exploration

Delve into the sensory aspects of eating with heightened awareness. Explore the textures, tastes, and scents of each bite. Allow the experience to unfold slowly, savoring the intricate details of your meal. This sensory exploration can enhance your overall enjoyment and satisfaction. By incorporating mindful eating practices into your daily life, you not only elevate your relationship with food but also create a foundation for deeper intimacy. As you engage in the art of mindful eating, you invite a heightened awareness and appreciation into your life, fostering a connection that extends beyond the dining table and into the realms of your most intimate moments. Creating a comprehensive 30-day plant-based diet plan for men's sexual wellness involves incorporating nutrient-rich foods that support overall health and vitality. It's important to note that individual nutritional needs may vary, and consulting with a healthcare professional or nutritionist is advisable before making significant dietary changes. Here's a sample 30-day plant-based diet plan along with a table highlighting key nutrients and suggested food sources.

CHAPTER SEVEN

Spicing up the immune system with unripe pawpaw [papaya]

While the benefits of unripe pawpaw (papaya) for plant-based potency in men aged 40-65 may not be extensively studied, there are some potential advantages associated with the consumption of this fruit. It's important to note that individual responses to dietary changes can vary, and consulting with a healthcare professional is recommended before making significant changes to one's diet. That said, here are some potential benefits of unripe pawpaw for men in this age group.

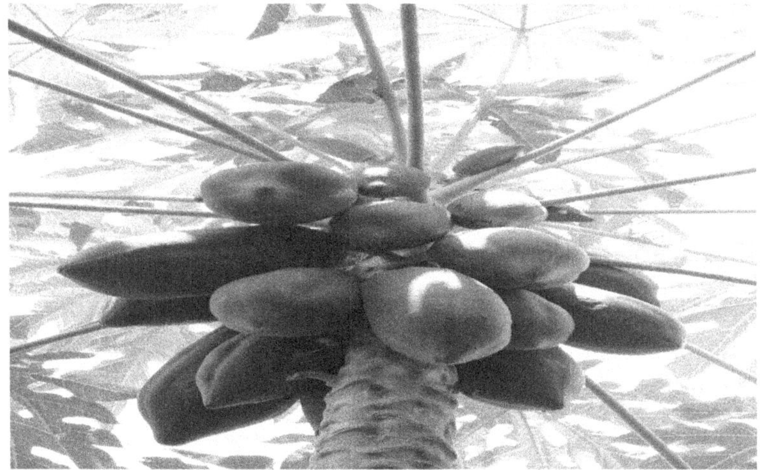

1.Rich in Nutrients

Unripe pawpaw is a good source of essential nutrients, including vitamins A, C, E, and folate. These vitamins play crucial roles in supporting overall health, including reproductive health.

2.Enzyme Papain

Unripe pawpaw contains an enzyme called papain, which is known for its digestive properties. A healthy digestive system is essential for nutrient absorption, and optimal nutrient levels can contribute to overall well-being.

3. Prostate Health

Some studies suggest that certain compounds found in pawpaw may have potential benefits for prostate health. Prostate issues become more prevalent as men age, and maintaining a healthy prostate is crucial for overall well-being.

4. Anti-Inflammatory Properties

Unripe pawpaw contains anti-inflammatory compounds, which may contribute to a reduction in inflammation within the body. Chronic inflammation is linked to various health issues, including those that may impact sexual health.

5. Rich in Antioxidants

Antioxidants found in unripe pawpaw, such as beta-carotene, help combat oxidative stress in the body. Oxidative stress has been linked to aging and age-related diseases, and reducing it may positively influence overall health.

6. Heart Health

A healthy cardiovascular system is vital for sexual health. Unripe pawpaw may contribute to heart health by supporting healthy blood pressure levels and reducing cholesterol.

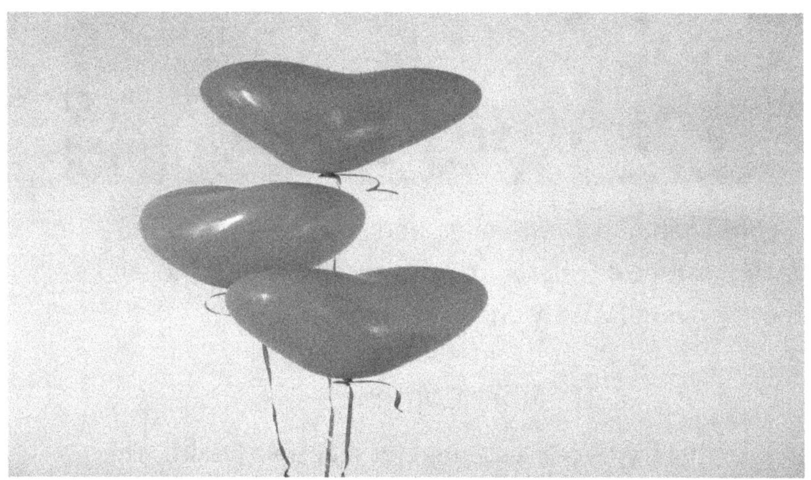

7. Blood Flow Improvement

Certain nutrients in unripe pawpaw may promote better blood circulation. Improved blood flow is crucial for sexual function and may help address issues related to potency.

8. Boosting Immunity

The rich content of vitamin C in unripe pawpaw supports the immune system. A robust immune system is important for overall health and vitality.

9. Natural Energy Boost

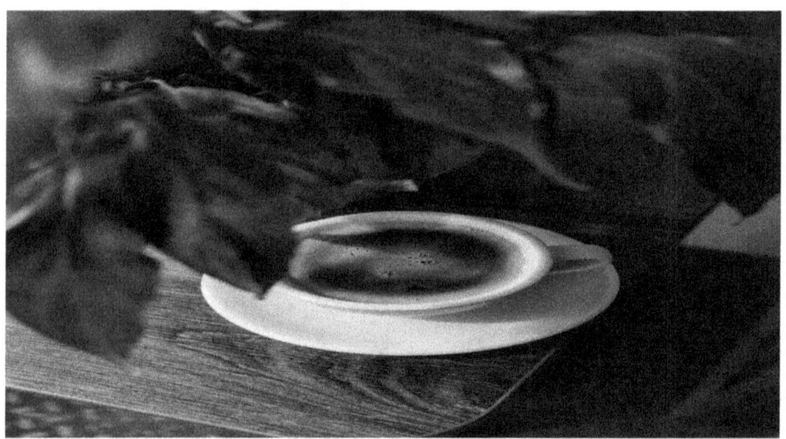

The combination of vitamins and minerals in unripe pawpaw can contribute to increased energy levels, promoting overall vitality and well-being.

10. Fiber Content

Adequate dietary fiber is essential for digestive health. The fiber in unripe pawpaw can support a healthy gut, promoting the absorption of nutrients critical for overall health.

While unripe pawpaw has potential health benefits, it's crucial to consume it as part of a balanced and varied diet.

Additionally, individual responses to dietary changes can vary, so consulting with a healthcare professional is advisable, especially for individuals with existing health conditions or those taking medications.

A balanced and nutritious diet cookbook for men age after 50 incorporating pawpaw can contribute to overall health and well-being. Here's a categorical breakdown of a basic diet including pawpaw

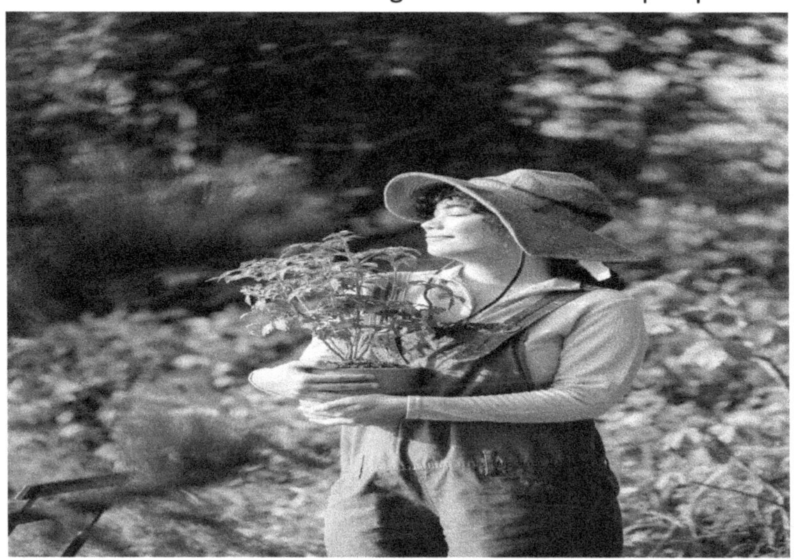

Harnessing Plant-Based for Optimal Potency

In this chapter our exploration into the realm of plant-based power, we delve into the profound impact that plant-based diets can have on human potency and overall well-being. As we navigate through the intricacies of nutrition, lifestyle, and the symbiotic relationship between plants and human health, we uncover the keys to unlocking optimal potency through plant-powered living.

Section 1 The Nutritional Foundations of Potency

1.1 Plant-Based Nutrients: A Potent Elixir

Explore the rich array of nutrients found in plant-based foods, including vitamins, minerals, antioxidants, and phytochemicals, and their role in supporting overall health and vitality. Highlight the synergistic effects of combining various plant-based sources to create a well-rounded and potent nutritional profile.

1.2 Plant Proteins and Performance

Examine the role of plant proteins in supporting muscle strength, endurance, and recovery.

Showcase the versatility of plant-based protein sources and dispel myths surrounding protein adequacy in plant-based diets.

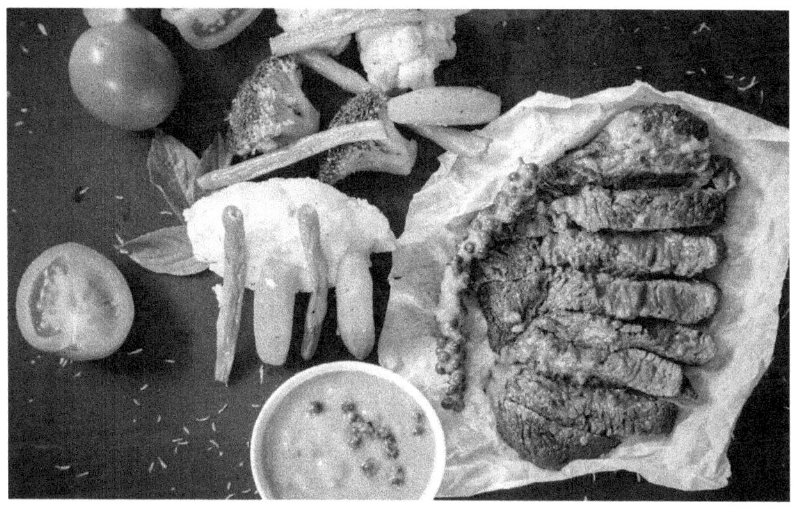

Section 2 Potency Beyond the Plate

2.1 Lifestyle Factors Cultivating Potency

Discuss the importance of lifestyle factors such as physical activity, adequate sleep, and stress management in enhancing overall potency. Showcase how adopting a plant-based lifestyle complements these factors to amplify their positive effects.

2.2 Mind-Body Connection: Mental Potency

Explore the connection between plant-based nutrition and mental well-being, including cognitive function, mood, and emotional resilience. Highlight studies demonstrating the positive impact of plant-based diets on mental health.

Section 3 Environmental Harmony and Potency

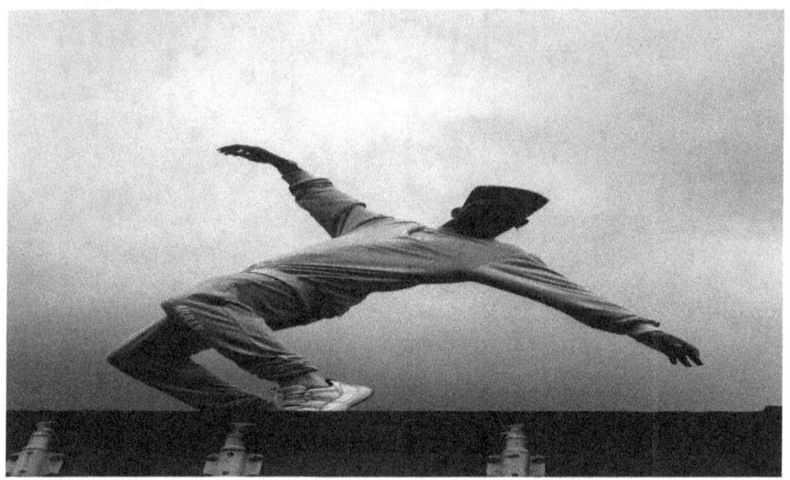

3.1 Sustainable Nutrition A Potent Force for the Planet

Discuss the environmental impact of plant-based diets compared to traditional animal-based diets. Emphasize the role of conscious eating in contributing to environmental sustainability and the preservation of natural resources.

3.2 Ethical Considerations Potency in Compassion

Address the ethical dimensions of plant-based living, including animal welfare and the compassionate choices individuals can make to align their values with their dietary habits.

CHAPTER EIGHT

Beverages and Refreshments

Collection of plant-based beverage recipes suitable for seniors, including herbal teas, infused waters, fruit juices, and smoothie variations. Tips for staying hydrated and incorporating hydrating beverages into daily routines. Suggestions for beverages to accompany meals or enjoy as snacks

Holiday and Special Occasion Menus

Compilation of plant-based recipes for festive occasions, celebrations, and special gatherings Ideas for creating holiday menus featuring traditional dishes adapted to be plant-based Tips for accommodating dietary restrictions and preferences of guests when hosting events

Seasonal and Local Produce

Overview of the benefits of consuming seasonal and local grown produce and guide to incorporating seasonal fruits, vegetables, and herbs into plant-based meals.

Tips for sourcing fresh, seasonal ingredients from farmers' markets, community-supported agriculture (CSA) programs, and local grocery stores

International Cuisine

Exploration of plant-based dishes from diverse culinary traditions around the world. Recipes for Mediterranean,

Asian, Latin American, Middle Eastern, and other international cuisines adapted to be plant-based. Information on unique ingredients and flavor profiles used in different cuisines.

Quick and Easy Meals for Busy Seniors

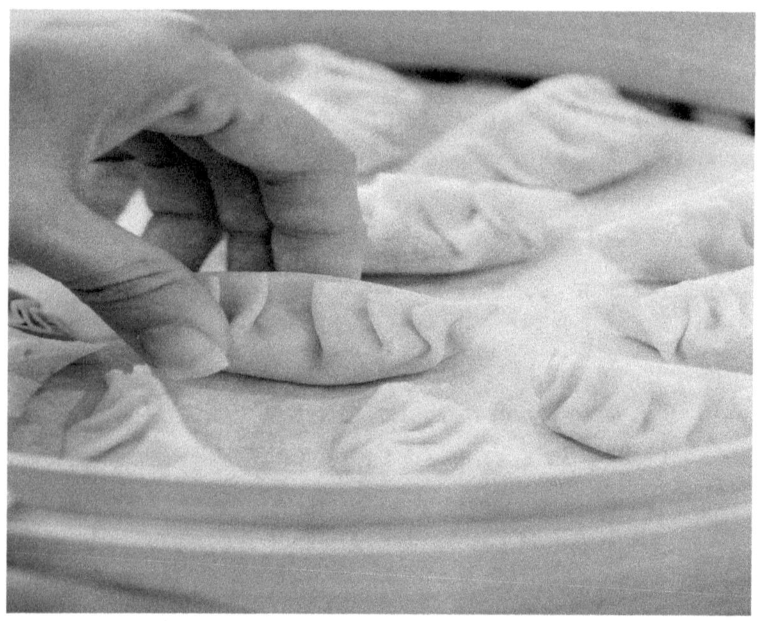

Collection of plant-based recipes designed for convenience and simplicity, perfect for seniors with busy lifestyles or limited time for cooking Recipes for one-pot meals, sheet pan dinners, 30-minute recipes, and make-ahead dishes. Tips for meal prep and batch cooking to streamline mealtime preparation.

Healthy Eating on a Budget

Strategies for seniors on a budget to incorporate more plant-based foods into their diet without breaking the bank Tips for saving money on groceries, such as buying in bulk, shopping sales, and minimizing food waste and recipes for budget-friendly plant-based meals and pantry staples.

Cooking for One or Two

Tips and recipes tailored to seniors who live alone or with a partner Ideas for adapting portion sizes and recipes to accommodate smaller households Strategies for reducing food waste when cooking for fewer people

Eating Out and Socializing

Guidance for seniors on navigating social situations and dining out while following a plant-based diet tips for finding plant-based options at restaurants, cafes, and social gatherings. Suggestions for communicating dietary preferences and restrictions to hosts and restaurant staff

Food Safety and Storage

Overview of best practices for food safety and storage to prevent foodborne illness tips for safely handling, storing, and reheating plant-based foods and Information on proper storage containers and labeling for leftovers and pantry items

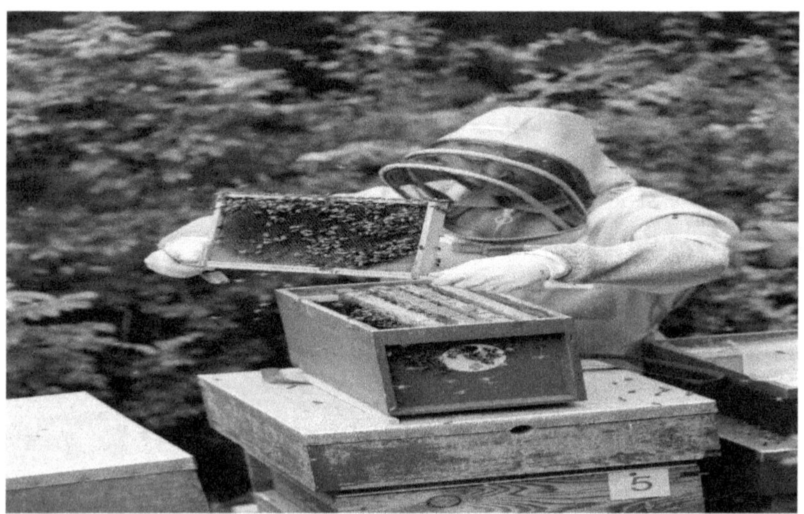

CHAPTER NINE

Staying Healthy and Active

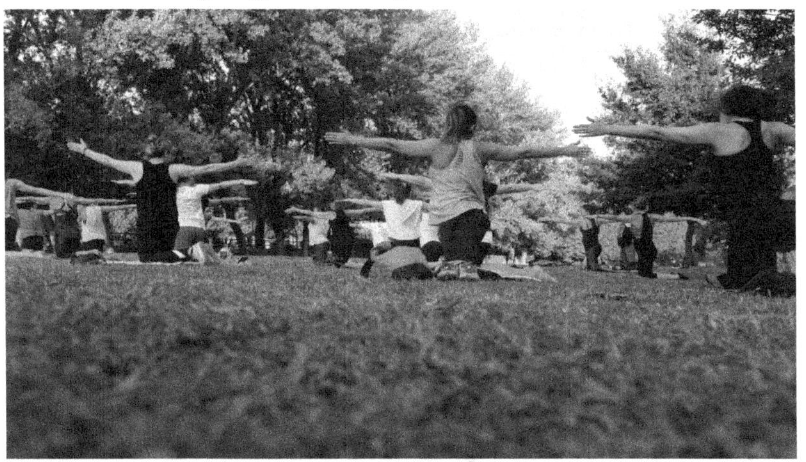

Discussion on the importance of maintaining a healthy lifestyle beyond diet for overall well-being in seniors and tips for staying physically active and incorporating movement into daily routines Suggestions for managing stress, getting adequate sleep, and fostering social connections for optimal health in older adults. This chapter would offer a combination of practical advice, culinary inspiration, and delicious recipes to support seniors in embracing a plant-based diet while promoting health, wellness, and enjoyment of food.

Mindful Eating Practices

Introduction to mindful eating techniques for seniors to cultivate a deeper connection with their food and tips for slowing down, savoring each bite, and paying attention to hunger and fullness cues. Guidance on mindful eating exercises to enhance enjoyment and appreciation of meals

Gardening and Homegrown Produce

Overview of the benefits of gardening for seniors, including physical activity, stress reduction, and access to fresh produce with tips for starting a garden, selecting suitable plants, and maintaining a garden space and the Ideas for incorporating homegrown fruits, vegetables, and herbs into plant-based meals

Food Allergies and Intolerances

Discussion on common food allergies and intolerances that may affect seniors. Guidance on identifying and avoiding allergens in plant-based recipes. Tips for substituting ingredients to accommodate dietary restrictions and preferences

Cooking with Herbs and Spices

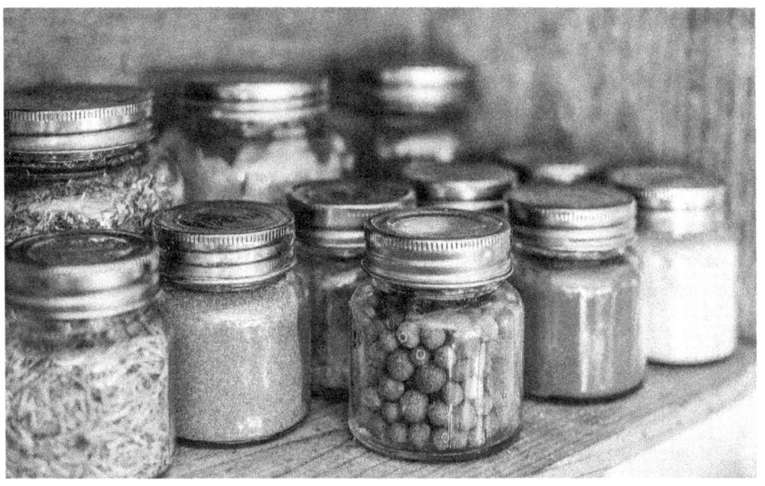

Exploration of the culinary uses and health benefits of herbs and spices in plant-based cooking. Guide to selecting, storing, and using a variety of herbs and spices to enhance flavor in recipes showcasing different herb and spice combinations for flavorful plant-based meals

Plant-Based Protein Sources

Overview of plant-based protein sources suitable for seniors, including legumes, tofu, tempeh, seitan, nuts, seeds, and whole grains for incorporating protein-rich foods into plant-based meals to support muscle health and overall well-being recipes highlighting different plant-based protein sources in satisfying and delicious dishes.

Fiber-Rich Foods and Digestive Health

Discussion on the importance of fiber for digestive health and regularity in seniors and guide to incorporating fiber-rich foods such as fruits, vegetables, whole grains, legumes, and nuts and seeds into the diet for preventing and managing common digestive issues through dietary strategies

Healthy Fats and Heart Health

Overview of the role of healthy fats in supporting heart health and overall well-being in seniors by incorporating sources of healthy fats such as avocados, nuts, seeds, and olive oil into a plant-based diet and the recipes featuring heart-healthy ingredients and cooking methods to promote cardiovascular health.

Sugar-Free and Low-Sugar Recipes

Collection of plant-based recipes with reduced or no added sugars, suitable for seniors with diabetes or those looking to reduce sugar intake with the tips for sweetening recipes naturally with fruit, dates, and other whole food ingredients including Ideas for satisfying sweet cravings without relying on refined sugars

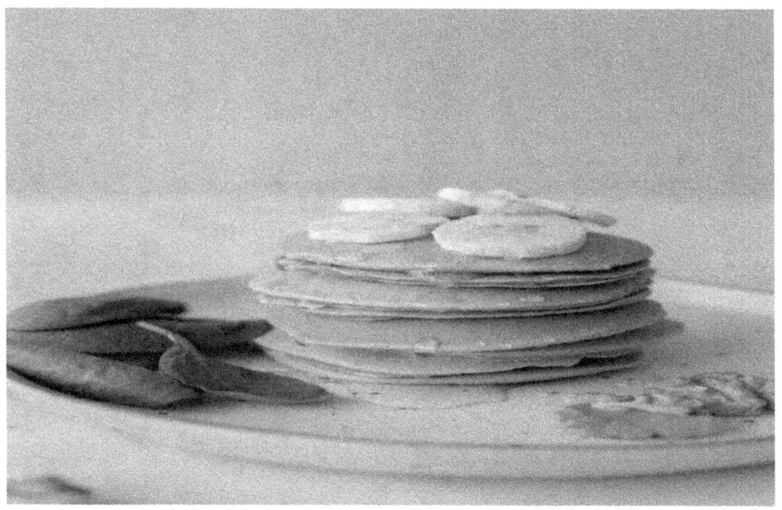

Gluten-Free and Grain-Free Options

Guide to gluten-free and grain-free alternatives for seniors with celiac disease, gluten sensitivity, or other dietary preferences recipes featuring gluten-free grains such as quinoa, rice, and millet, as well as grain-free options like cauliflower rice and spiralized vegetables for adapting recipes to be gluten-free or grain-free without sacrificing flavor or texture

Dairy-Free and Lactose-Free Recipes

Collection of plant-based recipes free from dairy and lactose, suitable for seniors with lactose intolerance or dairy allergies for substituting dairy ingredients with plant-based alternatives such as nut milks, coconut yogurt, and cashew cheese recipes for dairy-free versions of classic favorites like creamy soups, sauces, and desserts

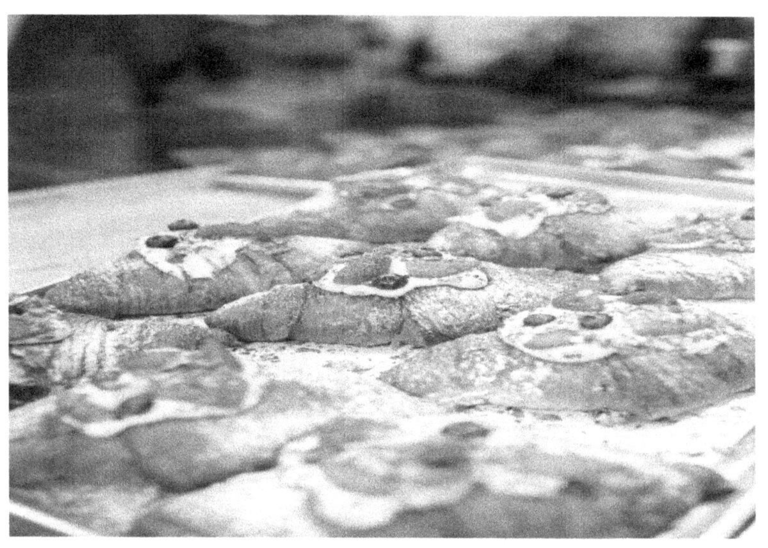

CHAPTER TEN

Cooking for Specific Dietary Needs

Guidance on cooking for seniors with specific dietary needs, including vegan, vegetarian, paleo, keto, and low-sodium diets for adapting recipes and meal plans to accommodate different dietary preferences and restrictions with recipes tailored to specific dietary patterns to support optimal health and well-being

Superfoods and Nutrient-Dense Ingredients

Exploration of nutrient-dense superfoods and ingredients that offer exceptional health benefits for seniors guide to incorporating superfoods such as berries, leafy greens, nuts, seeds, and seaweed into plant-based meals recipes featuring superfoods in delicious and nourishing dishes

Batch Cooking and Freezer-Friendly Meals.

Strategies for batch cooking and preparing freezer-friendly meals to save time and effort in the kitchen tips for safely storing and reheating batch-cooked meals for convenient and nutritious eating throughout the week and the recipes suitable for batch cooking and freezer storage, including soups, stews, casseroles, and grain-based dishes

Eating Well on the Go

Tips and recipes for seniors to maintain a plant-based diet while traveling, dining out, or eating away from home and ideas for portable snacks, pre-packaged meal options, and restaurant choices that align with a plant-based lifestyle. Suggestions for planning ahead and staying mindful of nutritional needs while on the go

Cooking with Family and Grandchildren

Healthy Aging and Longevity discussion on the role of diet and lifestyle factors in promoting healthy aging and longevity tips for seniors to adopt healthy habits such as regular physical activity, stress management, and social engagement recipes featuring nutrient-rich ingredients and anti-inflammatory foods to support overall health and well-being in later life

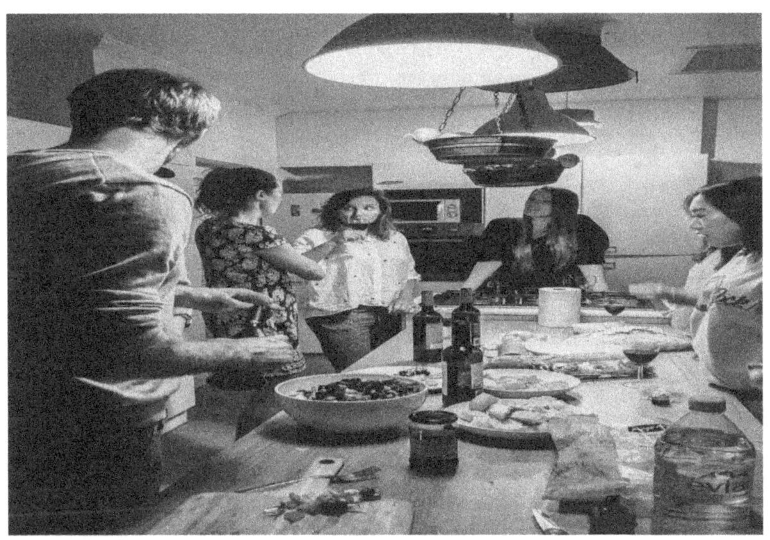

Mealtime Etiquette and Dining Alone

Guidance on maintaining enjoyable and meaningful mealtime experiences for seniors dining alone for setting a pleasant table, creating ambiance, and savoring meals mindfully ideas for staying connected with loved ones and creating virtual dining experiences

Kitchen Safety for Seniors

Overview of kitchen safety considerations for older adults, including preventing falls, burns, and cuts

for an organizing kitchen spaces for ease of use and accessibility, recommendations for using kitchen tools and appliances safely to minimize risk of injury

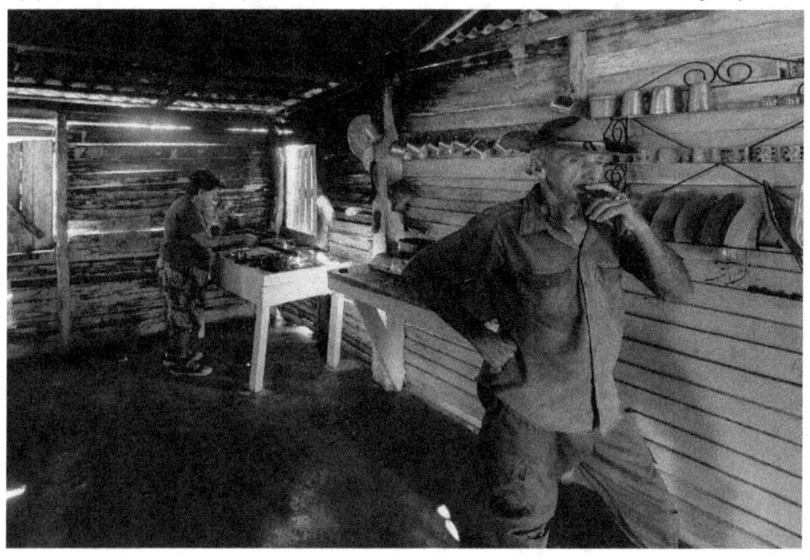

Cooking with Cognitive Impairment

Strategies for seniors with cognitive impairment to continue cooking and preparing meals safely and independently for simplifying recipes, using visual aids, and creating step-by-step instructions for engaging caregivers or family members in meal preparation and supervision

Eating Well with Chronic Health Conditions

Discussion on dietary strategies to manage common chronic health conditions in seniors, such as diabetes, heart disease, arthritis, and dementia, tips for adapting recipes and meal plans to accommodate specific dietary needs and restrictions

Recipes featuring ingredients and cooking techniques beneficial for managing chronic health conditions

Plant-Based Cooking for Two

Tips and recipes tailored to seniors cooking for themselves and a partner or spouse. Ideas for planning meals, adjusting portion sizes, and coordinating cooking responsibilities as a couple. Recipes designed for two servings, promoting shared enjoyment of plant-based meals

Cooking for Arthritis and Mobility Issues

Guidance on adapting cooking techniques and kitchen tools for seniors with arthritis or mobility issues. Tips for reducing strain on joints, improving grip strength, and enhancing kitchen accessibility. Recipes featuring easy-to-handle ingredients and simplified cooking methods for seniors with limited mobility. Strategies for handling social situations and dining out as a senior on a plant-based diet. Tips for communicating dietary preferences and needs to friends, family, and caregivers. Ideas for advocating for plant-based options in social settings and fostering supportive relationships

Seasonal Meal Planning

Guide to seasonal meal planning for seniors to enjoy fresh, locally sourced produce year-round. Tips for incorporating seasonal fruits, vegetables, and herbs into seasonal menus and recipes. Recipes highlighting seasonal ingredients and flavors for each time of year

Celebrating Cultural Traditions

Exploration of plant-based versions of traditional cultural dishes from around the world and recipes for celebrating cultural holidays and traditions with plant-based twists on classic favorites tips for incorporating cultural heritage into plant-based meal planning and cooking.

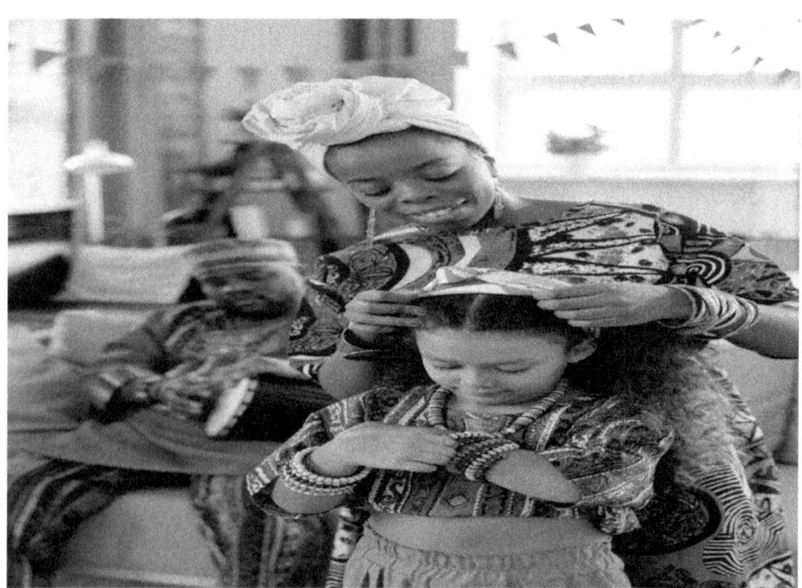

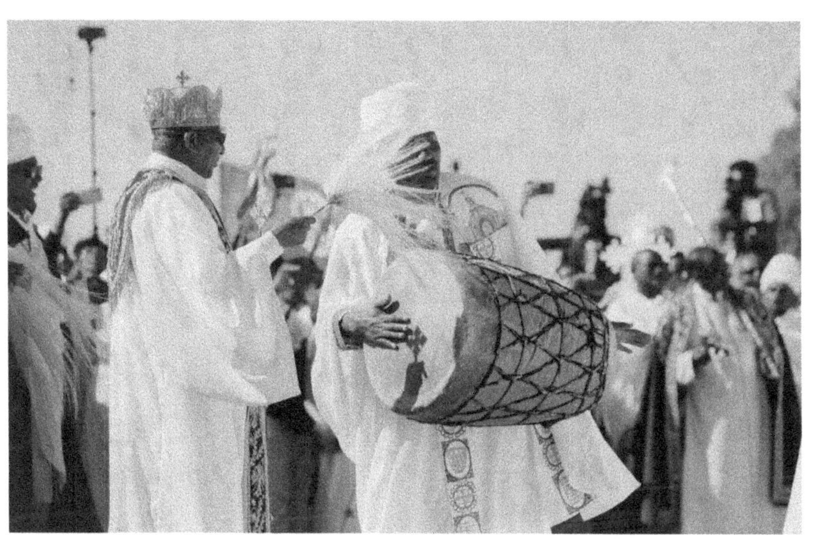

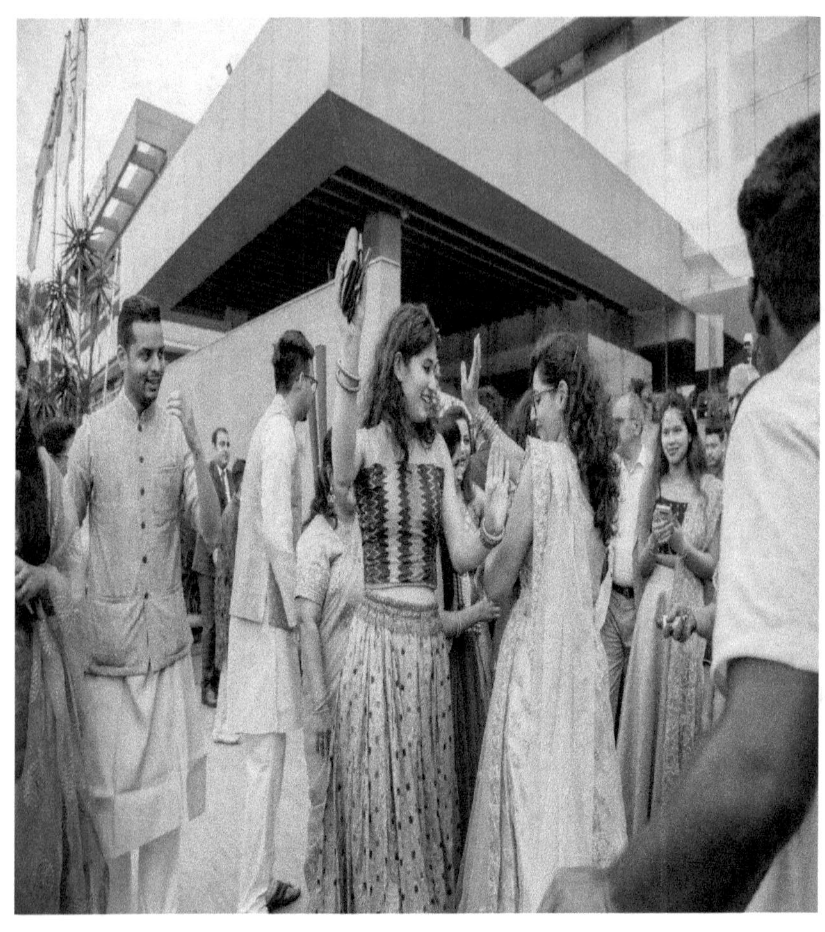

CHAPTER ELEVEN

Cooking for Heart Health

Recipes for seniors focused on maintaining heart health through diet and guidance on incorporating heart-healthy ingredients such as fruits, vegetables, whole grains, and lean plant-based proteins into meals, information on reducing sodium intake and minimizing added sugars and unhealthy fats in recipes

Plant-Based Picnics and Outdoor Dining

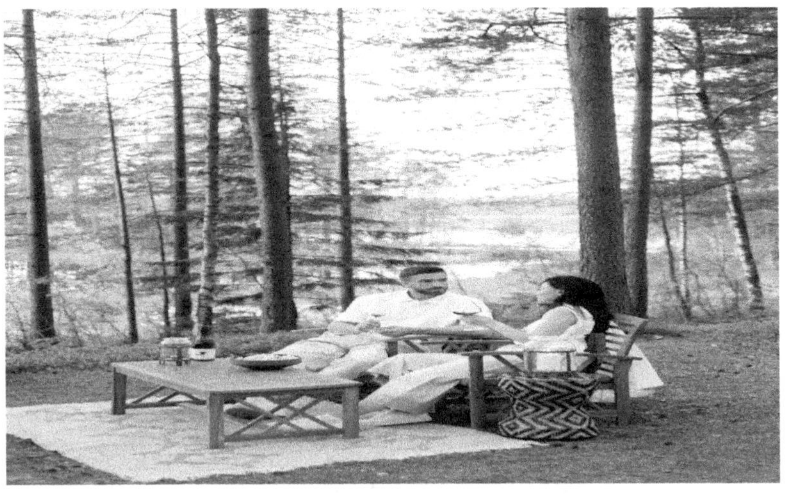

Ideas for planning and packing plant-based picnic meals for seniors to enjoy outdoors. Recipes for portable dishes, salads, sandwiches, and snacks suitable for picnics and

outdoor gatherings tips for staying safe and comfortable while dining al fresco

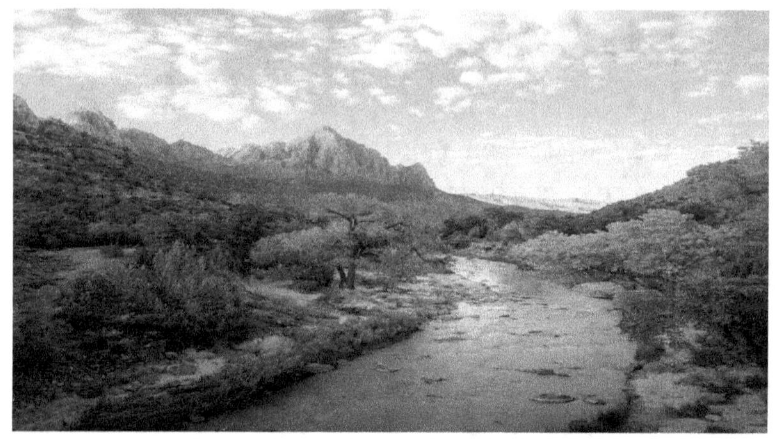

Mind-Body Wellness Practices

Introduction to mind-body wellness practices for seniors, such as meditation, yoga, and tai chi and tips for incorporating mindfulness and relaxation techniques into daily routines. Recipes featuring mood-boosting ingredients and stress-reducing foods to support overall well-being

Cooking with Limited Kitchen Facilities

Strategies for seniors with limited kitchen facilities, such as those living in assisted living facilities or nursing homes. Tips for making the most of available appliances and equipment, including microwave cooking and using small countertop appliances. Recipes requiring minimal cooking equipment and ingredients for easy preparation

Plant-Based Potluck Parties

Ideas for hosting and attending plant-based potluck parties with friends, family, and community members recipes for crowd-pleasing plant-based dishes suitable for sharing at potluck gatherings for coordinating potluck contributions, ensuring variety, and accommodating dietary preferences and restrictions

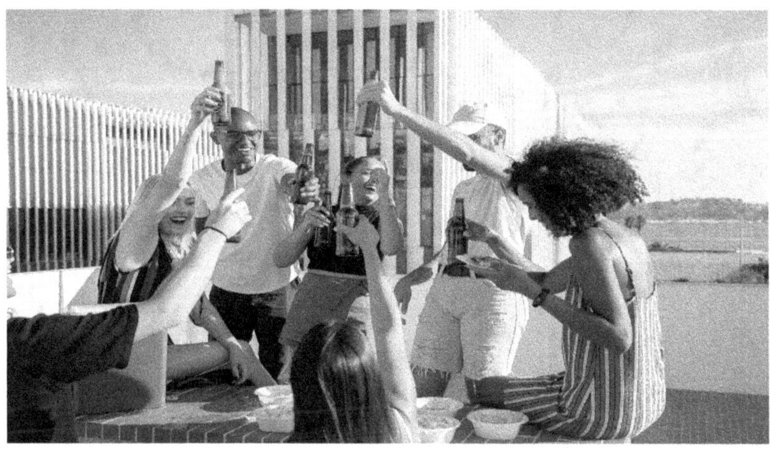

Cooking with Medicinal Herbs and Plants

Overview of culinary herbs and medicinal plants with potential health benefits for seniors and weight management

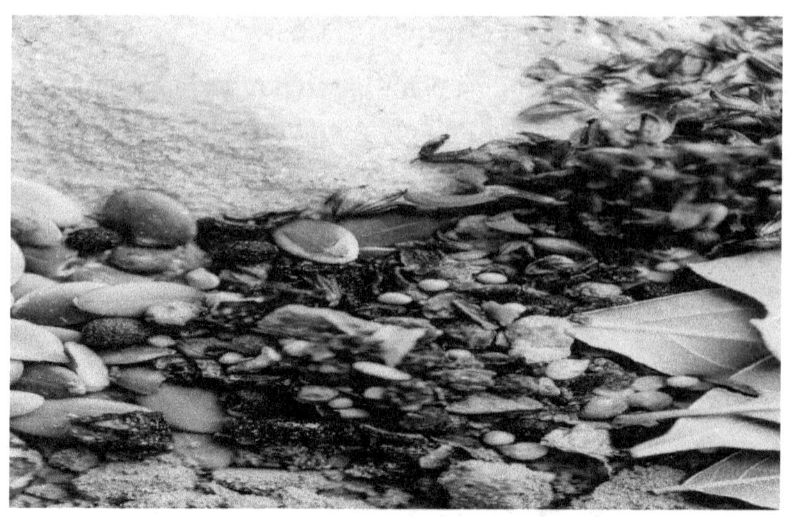

Recipes featuring herbs and plants known for their healing properties, such as ginger, turmeric, garlic, and echinacea and incorporating medicinal herbs and plants into everyday cooking for enhanced flavor and wellness and recipes for seniors focused on achieving and maintaining a healthy weight through diet. Guidance on portion control, mindful eating, and balancing macronutrients for weight management with recipes featuring low-calorie, nutrient-dense ingredients to support weight loss or weight maintenance goals

Plant-Based Holiday Feasts

Creating festive plant-based holiday menus for thanksgiving, Christmas, Hanukkah, Easter, and other celebrations also Recipes for holiday classics with plant-based twists, such as stuffed squash, lentil loaf, roasted vegetables, and dairy-free desserts and planning ahead, delegating tasks, accommodating guests' dietary preferences during holiday gatherings and cooking with canned and shelf-stable Foods. Strategies for seniors to utilize canned and shelf-stable foods in plant-based cooking and selecting nutritious canned goods and pantry staples, such as beans, tomatoes, coconut milk, and whole grains. Recipes featuring canned and shelf-stable ingredients for quick and convenient meal preparation

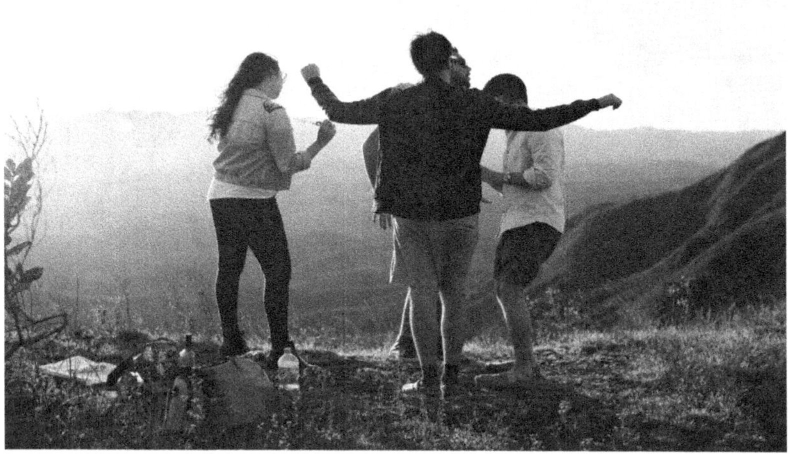

Plant-Based Camping Meals

Planning and preparing plant-based meals for camping trips and outdoor adventures with recipes for easy-to-pack camping meals, snacks, and treats suitable for cooking over a campfire or portable stove storing and transporting ingredients, minimizing waste, and practicing Leave No Trace principles while camping

Cooking with Fresh Herbs and Edible Flowers

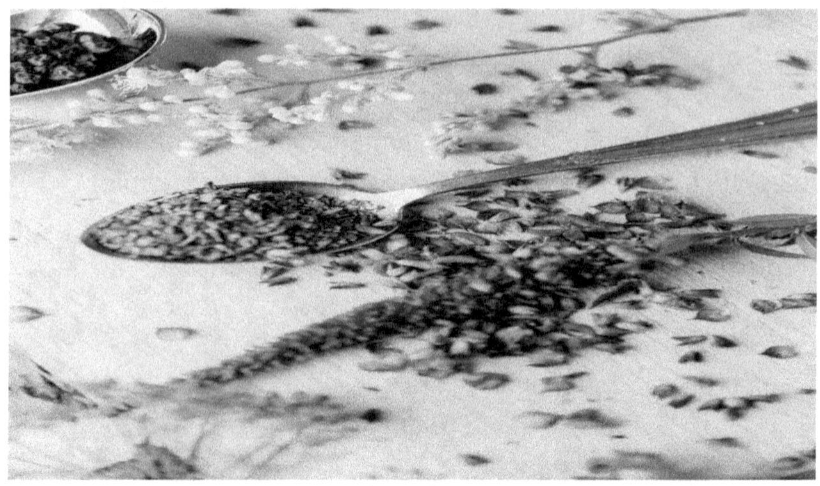

Guide to using fresh herbs and edible flowers to enhance the flavor, aroma, and presentation of plant-based dishes. Tips for growing and harvesting herbs and flowers at home or purchasing them from farmers' markets and specialty stores. Recipes featuring fresh herbs and edible flowers in salads, dressings, sauces, and desserts

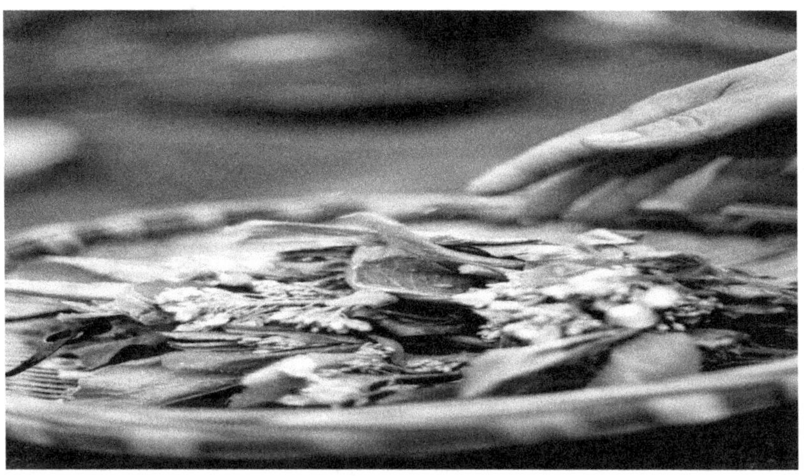

Cooking for Bone Health

Recipes and tips for seniors focused on supporting bone health through diet. Guidance on incorporating calcium-rich plant foods such as leafy greens, tofu, almonds, and fortified plant milks into meals Information on vitamin D sources, magnesium, and other nutrients important for bone health

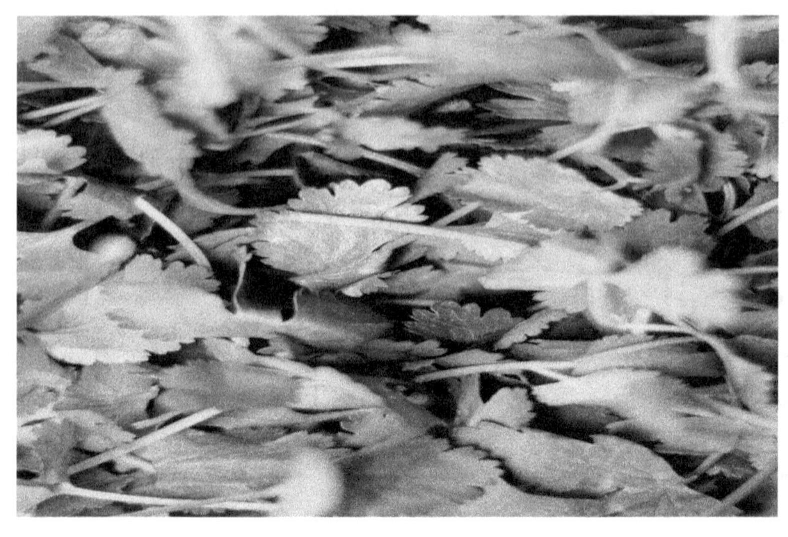

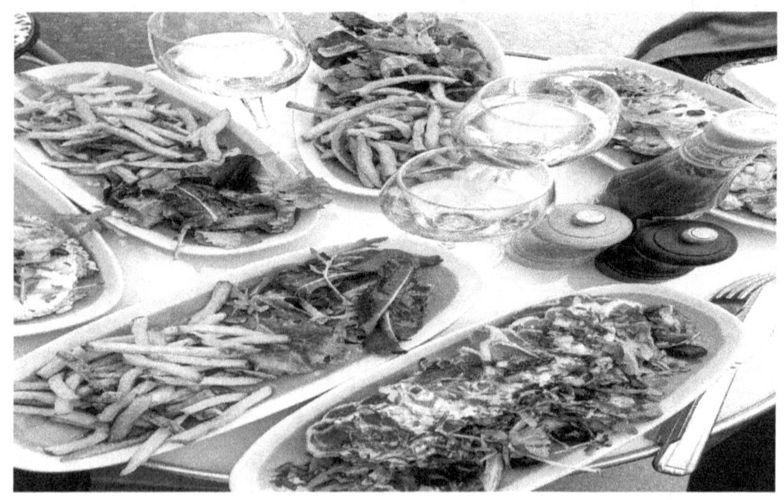

CHAPTER TWELVE

Plant-Based Breakfasts on the Go

Ideas and recipes for quick and portable plant-based breakfast options for busy mornings

Recipes for grab-and-go breakfasts, make-ahead meals, and portable snacks suitable for eating on the go for balancing convenience, nutrition, and flavor in breakfasts for seniors with busy schedules

Cooking for Respiratory Health

Recipes and tips for seniors focused on supporting respiratory health through diet. Guidance and incorporating Anti-inflammatory foods, immune-boosting nutrients,and respiratory-supportive herbs into meals.

Information on foods and nutrients that may help manage respiratory conditions such as asthma, COPD, and allergies

Plant-Based Entertaining and Hosting

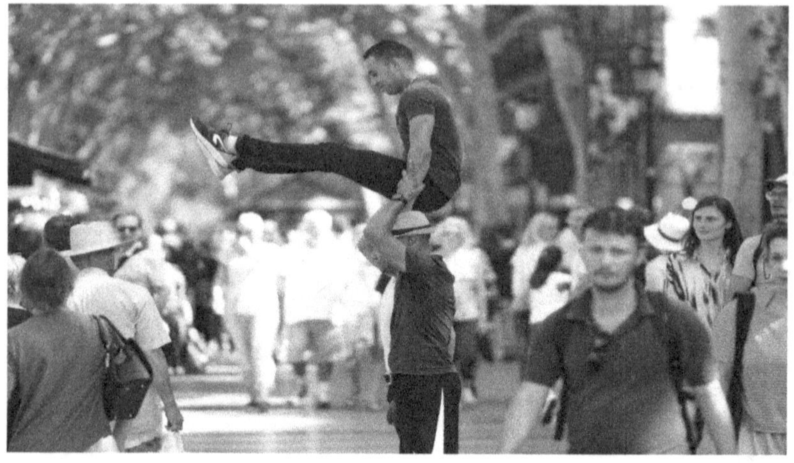

Ideas for hosting plant-based gatherings and entertaining guests at home

Recipes for impressive plant-based appetizers, mains, sides, and desserts suitable for special occasions and celebrations

Tips for planning menus, decorating, and creating a welcoming atmosphere for guests

Cooking with Fermented Foods and Comfort

Introduction to fermented foods and their potential health benefits for seniorsGuide to incorporating fermented foods such as sauerkraut, kimchi, tempeh, and miso into plant-based meals. Recipes featuring fermented ingredients and condiments for added flavor and gut health support for satisfying and nourishing plant-based comfort foods reminiscent of familiar favorites ideas for creating plant-based versions of classic comfort dishes such as macaroni and cheese, shepherd's pie, lasagna, and creamy soups for using comforting flavors and textures to create satisfying plant-based meals for seniors

Cooking for Vision Health

Recipes and tips for seniors focused on supporting vision health through diet. Guidance on incorporating antioxidant-rich foods, omega-3 fatty acids, and eye-friendly nutrients into meals. Information on foods and nutrients that may help protect against age-related eye conditions such as macular degeneration and cataracts

Plant-Based Grilling and Barbecue

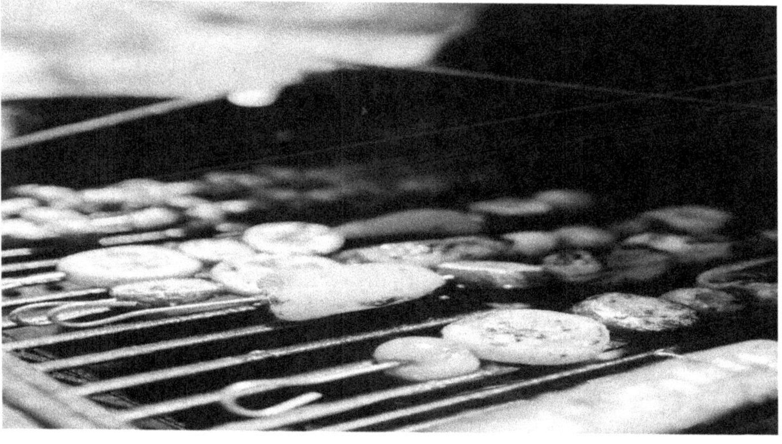

Ideas and recipes for plant-based grilling and barbecue parties with friends and family recipes for grilled vegetables, plant-based burgers, kebabs, skewers, and barbecue sauces and marinades

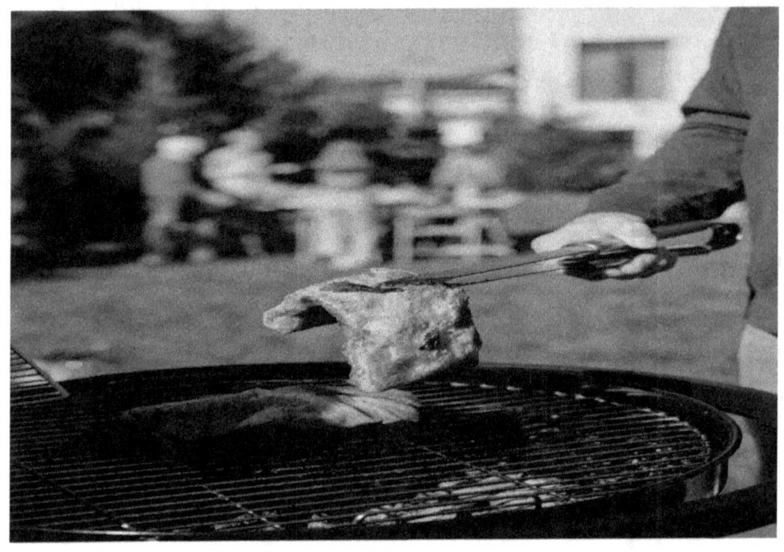

Tips for preparing and cooking plant-based foods on the grill for optimal flavor and texture cooking with Whole Grains. Guide to cooking with a variety of whole grains such as quinoa, brown rice, barley, farro, and bulgur recipes featuring whole grains as the star ingredient in salads, pilafs, grain bowls, soups, and baked goods for selecting, storing, and cooking whole grains for maximum flavor and nutritional value with high-Protein Recipes Recipes and tips for seniors focused on increasing protein intake through plant-based sources. Guidance on protein-rich foods such as beans, lentils, tofu, tempeh, and seitan into meals. Information on protein requirements for seniors and the importance of protein for muscle health and overall well-being. Cooking for digestive health recipes and tips for seniors focused on supporting digestive health through diet. Incorporating fiber-rich foods, probiotics, and gut-friendly nutrients into meals information on foods and nutrients that may help manage digestive issues such as constipation, bloating, and irritable bowel syndrome.

Plant-Based Slow Cooking

Ideas and recipes for plant-based slow cooker meals for seniors looking for easy, hands-off cooking solutions for hearty soups, stews, chilis, curries, and braises designed for slow cooking, adapting recipes and using slow cookers safely and effectively for plant-based cooking for Brain Health for seniors focused on supporting brain health through diet, guidance on incorporating brain-boosting foods such as leafy greens, berries, nuts, seeds, and omega-3 fatty acids into meals

The information on foods and nutrients that may help protect against cognitive decline and support overall brain function with a comprehensive exploration of different aspects of plant-based cooking tailored specifically for seniors, offering practical advice, culinary inspiration, and delicious recipes to support their health, well-being, and enjoyment of food.

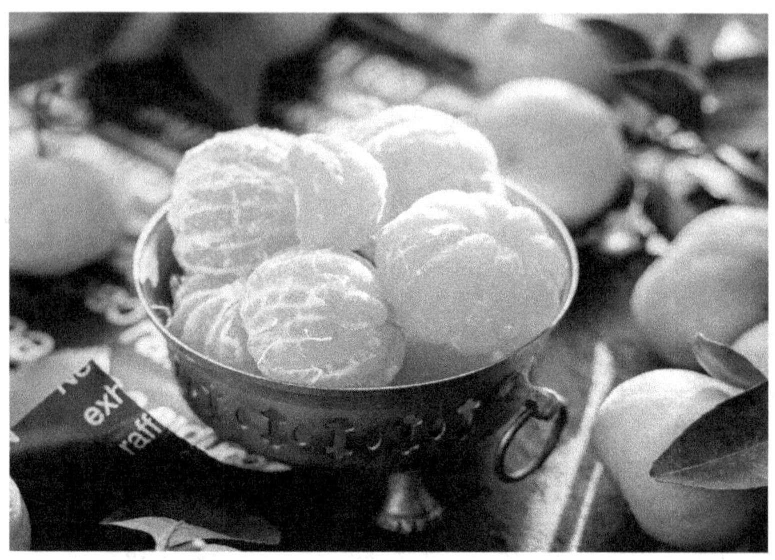

Cooking for Joint Health

Recipes and tips for seniors focused on supporting joint health through diet guidance on anti-inflammatory foods, omega-3 fatty acids, and joint-supportive nutrients into meals and Information on foods and nutrients that may help reduce joint pain and inflammation associated with conditions such as arthritis

Cooking for Immune Support

Recipes and tips for seniors focused on supporting immune health through diet.

Guidance on incorporating immune-boosting foods, antioxidants, and vitamins and minerals into meals

Information on foods and nutrients that may help strengthen the immune system and protect against illness with budget-friendly ingredients strategies and recipes for seniors on a budget to prepare nutritious and delicious plant-based meals without overspending Guidance on shopping smart, buying in bulk, and making the most of affordable ingredients such as beans, lentils, grains, and seasonal produce and tips for meal planning, batch cooking, and minimizing food waste to stretch the food budget further

Healthy Skin

Recipes for seniors focused on promoting healthy skin through diet

Guidance on incorporating skin-nourishing foods such as fruits, vegetables, nuts, seeds, and omega-3 fatty acids into meals

Information on foods and nutrients that may help maintain skin elasticity, hydration, and overall appearance

Dental Health

Recipes and tips for seniors focused on supporting dental health through diet

Guidance on incorporating tooth-friendly foods such as crunchy fruits and vegetables, calcium-rich foods, and vitamin C-rich foods into meals

Information on foods and nutrients that may help prevent tooth decay, gum disease, and other oral health issues

Fermented Beverages

Ideas and recipes for homemade fermented beverages packed with probiotics and other beneficial nutrients recipes for kombucha, water kefir Ideas for involving family members, including grandchildren, In plant-based cooking and meal preparation tips for creating positive cooking experiences and fostering intergenerational connections in the kitchen. Each chapter provides a wealth of information, practical tips, and delicious recipes tailored to the needs and preferences of seniors adopting a plant-based diet. Together, these chapters aim to support older adults in embracing a healthier lifestyle and enjoying the benefits of plant-based eating.

Eye Health

Discussion on the importance of nutrition for maintaining eye health as we age. The overview of nutrients that support eye health, such as vitamin A, lutein, zeaxanthin, and omega-3 fatty acids, and their food sources recipes featuring ingredients rich in eye-friendly nutrients, including leafy greens, colorful fruits and vegetables, nuts, seeds, and fatty fish alternatives for eye-healthy foods into meals and snacks to support vision and prevent age-related eye conditions. Information on lifestyle factors that contribute to eye health, such as regular exercise, wearing sunglasses, and quitting smoking

Cooking for Gut Health

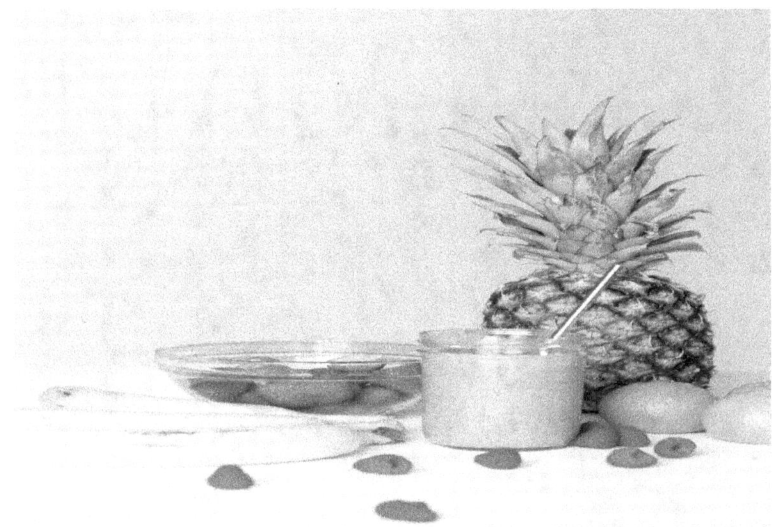

Overview of the gut microbiome and its role in overall health and well-being. Explanation of how diet influences gut health, including the importance of fiber, fermented foods, and prebiotics recipes featuring gut-friendly ingredients such as fiber-rich fruits and vegetables, fermented foods, whole grains, and legumes tips for incorporating gut-healthy foods into meals and snacks to support digestion, immune function, and mental healthInformation on lifestyle factors that promote gut health, including regular exercise, stress management, and adequate sleep. These book provide seniors with valuable information and practical tips for improving their health and well-being through plant-based cooking and nutrition. From fermented beverages to eye health, meal prep, and gut health, each chapter offers valuable insights and delicious recipes tailored to the unique needs of older adults.

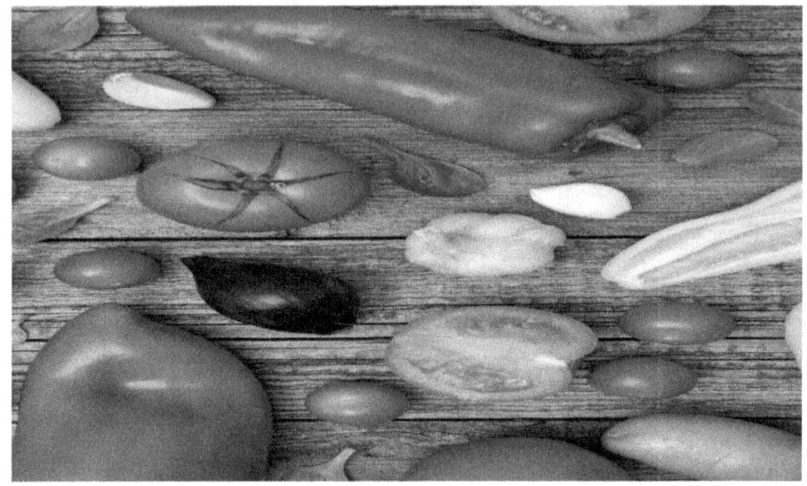

CONCLUSION

Cultivating Potency Through Plant-Based Power

Summarize the key insights from the exploration of plant-based power and its impact on potency. Encourage readers to consider the holistic approach of adopting a plant-based lifestyle for optimal health, environmental sustainability, and ethical considerations. Emphasize the idea that harnessing plant-based power is not just a dietary choice but a transformative journey towards a potent and harmonious existence.

Nutritional effects of pawpaw[papaya]

1.Breakfast

Pawpaw Smoothie

Blend unripe pawpaw with other fruits like bananas, berries, and a handful of spinach. Add a scoop of protein powder for an extra boost.

2.Whole Grain Toast

Top with avocado or nut butter for healthy fats and additional nutrients.

Greek Yogurt

High in protein and probiotics, Greek yogurt can be paired with a sprinkle of nuts or seeds.

3. Mid-Morning Snack

Pawpaw Slices

Enjoy fresh pawpaw slices as a snack, providing a dose of vitamins and natural sugars.

Handful of Almonds

A good source of healthy fats and vitamin E.

4. Lunch

Grilled Chicken Salad

Include pawpaw chunks in a mixed green salad with grilled chicken, cherry tomatoes, and a light vinaigrette dressing.

Quinoa Bowl

Combine cooked quinoa with vegetables, beans, and diced pawpaw for a nutrient-rich lunch.

Afternoon Snack

Pawpaw and Cottage Cheeses

Pair pawpaw slices with a serving of cottage cheese for a protein-rich snack.

Whole Grain Crackers

Enjoy with hummus or guacamole for added nutrients.

5. Dinner

Baked Fish or Lean Meat

Choose a lean protein source like fish or skinless poultry, and accompany it with a side of steamed vegetables and a small serving of pawpaw salsa.

Quinoa or Brown Rice

These whole grains provide fiber and essential nutrients.

Stir-Fried Vegetables

Include a variety of colorful vegetables for added vitamins and minerals.

6.Evening Snack [Optional]

Pawpaw and Greek Yogurt Parfait

Layer pawpaw chunks with Greek yogurt and a sprinkle of granola or nuts.

7. Hydration

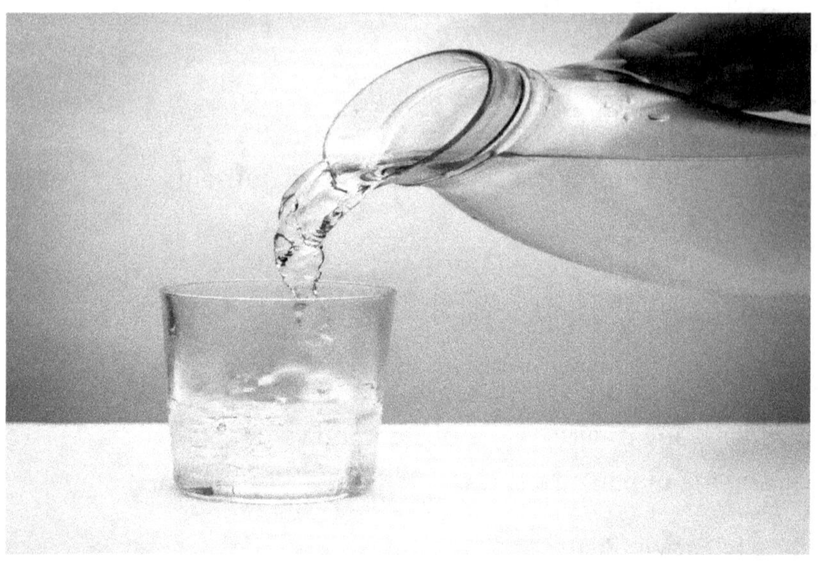

Water

Stay well-hydrated throughout the day by drinking plenty of water.

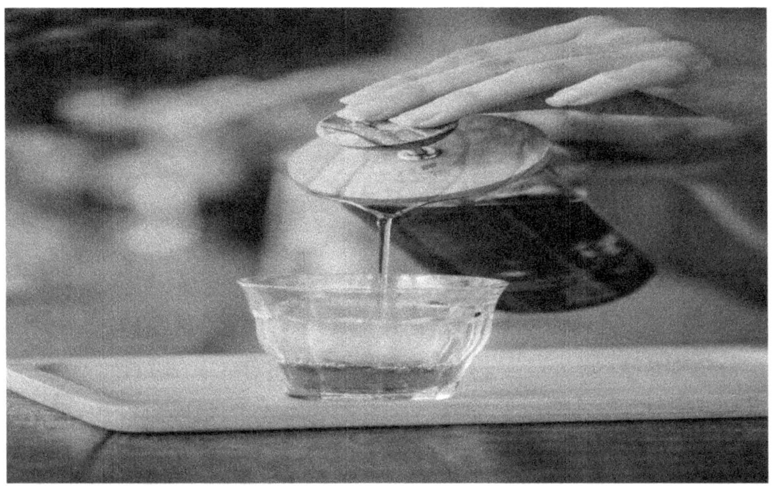

opt for caffeine-free herbal teas for added hydration. Remember, it's essential to maintain a varied and balanced diet that includes a mix of fruits, vegetables, lean proteins, whole grains, and healthy fats. While pawpaw can be a nutritious addition, it should be part of an overall healthy lifestyle. Additionally, individual dietary needs may vary, so consulting with a healthcare professional or a registered dietitian is recommended, especially for those with specific health concerns or conditions.

Key Nutrients and Their Sources

1. **Protein**: Lentils, chickpeas, tofu, tempeh, quinoa, nuts, seeds.
2. **Fiber:** Whole grains, fruits, vegetables, legumes, nuts, seeds.

3. **Omega**-3 Fatty Acids: Flaxseeds, chia seeds, walnuts, hemp seeds.
4. **Iron:** Lentils, spinach, quinoa, tofu, beans, fortified cereals.
5. **Zinc**: Beans, lentils, pumpkin seeds, cashews, quinoa.
6. **Vitamins (A, C, E, D, B12):** Dark leafy greens, fruits, nuts, seeds, fortified foods.
7. **Calcium:** Tofu, kale, book choy, fortified plant milk.
8. **Antioxidants:** Berries, tomatoes, dark chocolate, spinach, nuts.

Remember to stay hydrated, incorporate variety in your meals, and adjust portion sizes based on your individual needs. This plan aims to provide a diverse range of nutrients that can contribute to overall health and support men's sexual wellness.

Cultivating a Lifestyle of Diet Pleasure

As we conclude our exploration in "plant-based diet cookbook: A Culinary Guide to Men's Sexual Wellness," we find ourselves at the crossroads of nourishment and intimacy, where the vibrant world of plant-based nutrition intersects with the realms of desire, vitality, and overall well-being. The journey embarked upon has been a celebration of flavors, an unveiling of secrets hidden in nature's bounty, and an invitation to cultivate a lifestyle that harmonizes both body and intimacy.

In the quest for sexual wellness, we've traversed the landscapes of green aphrodisiacs, delving into the nutrient-rich embrace of leafy greens, avocados, and the oceanic potency of spirulina. We've sown the seeds of vigor, exploring the diverse contributions of chia seeds, pumpkin seeds, almonds, and others to male vitality and hormonal balance. The sweet sensations of fruits, from antioxidant-rich berries to exotic treasures like mangoes and pomegranates, have captivated our taste buds while contributing to improved blood flow and desire.

Spices became our allies in spicing up love lives, as saffron, cinnamon, ginger, cardamom, and vanilla infused our culinary creations with passion, warmth, and sensuality. The journey culminated in crafting elixirs of love — plant-powered beverages designed not only for refreshment but as companions in the pursuit of blissful nights. From floral infusions to energizing smoothies, each elixir became a celebration of plant-powered pleasure.

As we reflect on this culinary adventure, the conclusion is not just an end but a continuation of a lifestyle. Embracing plant-based diet cookbook is an ongoing commitment to prioritize well-being, savor the richness of nature's offerings, and nurture the intimate connections that define our human experience. The holistic approach advocated in these pages extends beyond the kitchen; it encompasses a mindset, a conscious choice to infuse every aspect of life with the vitality and pleasure derived from plant-powered nutrition.

So, as you step away from these pages, let them be a springboard for a lifestyle rich in plant-based pleasure, where every meal becomes a celebration of both health and desire. The keys to sexual wellness lie not just in the ingredients but in the intention, mindfulness, and joy infused into every culinary creation. May the knowledge gained here inspire you to continue exploring the boundless possibilities of plant-based living, cultivating a healthier, more vibrant life filled with the pleasures that nature so generously provides.

Cheers to a life where the pursuit of pleasure and well-being converges—a life truly powered by the potency of plants. vet becomes a celebration of plant-based pleasure.

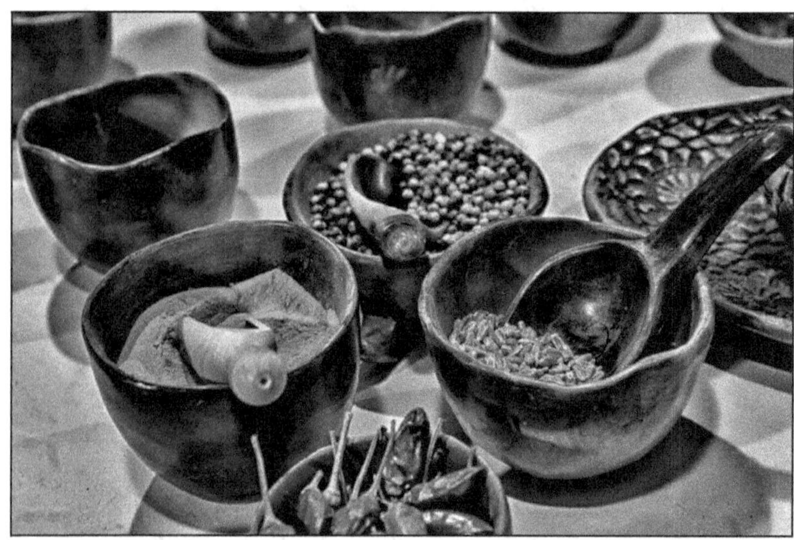

A 30-Day Diet Cookbook for Seniors

Welcome to "Nourishing Plant-Based Meals," a comprehensive 30-day cookbook designed specifically for seniors. This cookbook aims to provide delicious, nutritious, and easy-to-prepare plant-based recipes tailored to meet the unique dietary needs of older adults. Whether you're new to plant-based eating or a seasoned pro, this cookbook offers a variety of flavors and textures to keep your meals exciting and satisfying. With an emphasis on whole foods and nutrient-dense ingredients, each recipe is thoughtfully crafted to support overall health and well-being. Get ready to embark on a journey of vibrant flavors and wholesome eating that will leave you feeling energized and nourished.

Day 1 Breakfast
Creamy oatmeal topped with fresh berries, nuts, and a drizzle of maple syrup
Green smoothie with spinach, banana, almond milk, and a scoop of plant-based protein powder

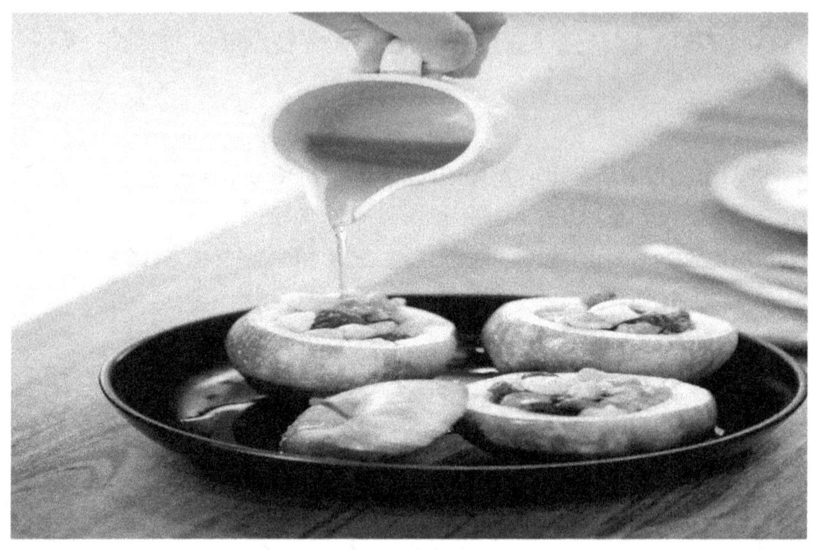

Day 2 Lunch

Chickpea salad sandwich with mashed chickpeas, diced vegetables, and vegan mayo on whole grain bread

Mixed greens salad with sliced avocado, cherry tomatoes, cucumber, and a balsamic vinaigrette dressing

Day 3 Dinner

Lentil and vegetable stew served with whole grain bread

Roasted Brussels sprouts and sweet potatoes seasoned with garlic and herbs

Day 4 Breakfast

Tofu scramble with sautéed vegetables (bell peppers, onions, spinach) and a side of whole grain toast

Fresh fruit salad with a sprinkle of chia seeds

Day 5 Lunch

Quinoa salad with roasted vegetables (zucchini, bell peppers, eggplant) and a lemon tahini dressing

Steamed broccoli with a squeeze of lemon and a sprinkle of nutritional yeast

Day 6 Dinner

Vegan chili loaded with beans, tomatoes, corn, and spices, served with a side of brown rice

Baked sweet potato topped with black beans, salsa, and avocado

Day 7 Breakfast

Whole grain pancakes topped with sliced bananas and a dollop of almond butter

Mixed berry smoothie with almond milk and a handful of spinach

Day 8 Lunch

Hummus and veggie wrap with shredded carrots, cucumber, lettuce, and hummus wrapped in a whole grain tortilla

Tomato basil soup served with a side of whole grain crackers

Day 9 Dinner

Stir-fried tofu and mixed vegetables (broccoli, bell peppers, snap peas) served over brown rice.

Steamed edamame sprinkled with sea salt

Day 10 Breakfast

Overnight chia seed pudding topped with sliced peaches and almonds

Whole grain toast with mashed avocado and cherry tomatoes

Day 11 Lunch

Mediterranean quinoa bowl with chickpeas, olives, cucumber, tomato, and a lemon tahini dressing

Roasted cauliflower florets seasoned with turmeric and cumin

Day 12 Dinner

Spaghetti squash with marinara sauce and vegan meatballs

Steamed green beans with garlic and lemon zest

Day 13 Breakfast

Smoothie bowl topped with granola, sliced strawberries, and shredded coconut

Whole grain English muffin with almond butter and sliced apple

Day 14 Lunch

Falafel salad with mixed greens, cucumber, tomato, olives, and a tahini dressing

Baked sweet potato fries with a sprinkle of paprika

Day 15 Dinner

Vegetable stir-fry with tofu, broccoli, bell peppers, carrots, and snap peas served over quinoa

Roasted beets with balsamic glaze

Day 16 Breakfast

Breakfast burrito with scrambled tofu, black beans, salsa, and avocado wrapped in a whole grain tortilla

Fresh fruit salad with a squeeze of lime juice

Day 17 Lunch

Lentil soup with diced vegetables and a side of whole grain bread

Mixed greens salad with roasted butternut squash, walnuts, and a balsamic vinaigrette dressing

Day 18 Dinner

Vegan shepherd's pie with lentils, mixed vegetables, and mashed sweet potatoes

Steamed asparagus with a drizzle of olive oil and lemon juice

Day 19 Breakfast

Coconut yogurt parfait with granola, mixed berries, and a drizzle of agave syrup

Whole grain toast with mashed avocado and sliced tomato

Day 20 Lunch

Black bean and corn salad with diced avocado, red onion, cilantro, and lime dressing

Roasted Brussels sprouts with a balsamic glaze

Day 21 Dinner

Stuffed bell peppers with quinoa, black beans, corn, and salsa

Sautéed spinach with garlic and pine nuts

Day 22 Breakfast

Smoothie with kale, banana, mango, and coconut water

Whole grain pancakes topped with sliced peaches and a sprinkle of cinnamon

Day 23 Lunch

Vegan sushi rolls with avocado, cucumber, carrot, and tofu

Miso soup with tofu and seaweed

Day 24 Dinner

Chickpea curry served with brown rice
Roasted root vegetables (carrots, parsnips, potatoes)
seasoned with rosemary and thyme

Day 25 Breakfast

Overnight oats with almond milk, chia seeds, and
mixed berries
Whole grain toast with almond butter and sliced
banana

Day 26 Lunch

Buddha bowl with quinoa, roasted sweet potato,
avocado, shredded kale, and tahini dressing
Grilled portobello mushrooms with balsamic glaze

Day 27 Dinner

Vegetable paella with bell peppers, peas, artichokes,
and saffron rice
Steamed broccoli with a squeeze of lemon

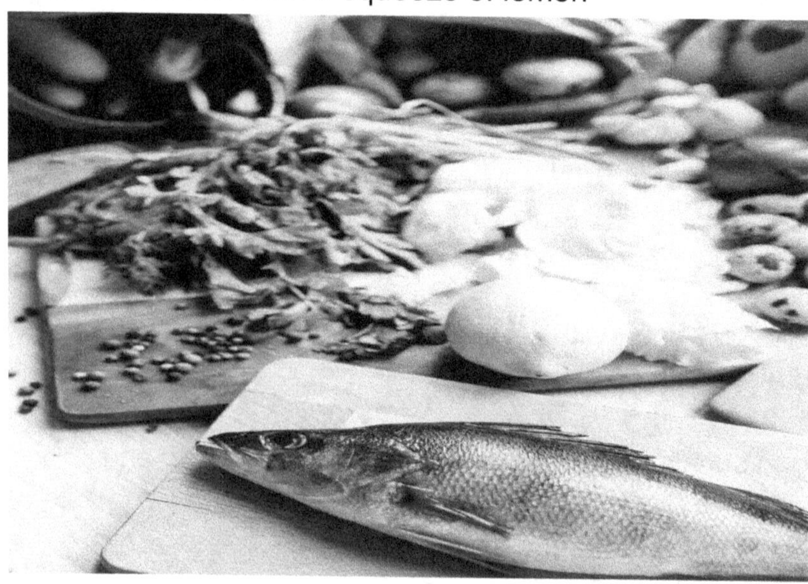

Day 28 Breakfast

Tofu scramble wrap with sautéed vegetables and salsa in a whole grain tortilla
Fresh fruit salad with a sprinkle of hemp seeds

Day 29 Lunch

Lentil salad with diced vegetables, parsley, and a lemon vinaigrette dressing
Baked potato topped with vegan chili and diced onions

Day 30 Dinner

Eggplant lasagna with layers of roasted eggplant, marinara sauce, and vegan ricotta cheese
Mixed greens salad with cherry tomatoes, cucumber, and a balsamic vinaigrette dressing

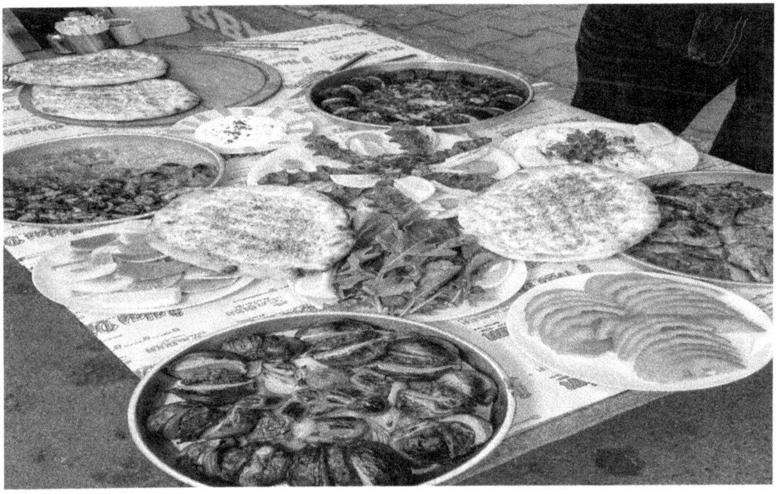

Congratulations on completing the "Nourishing Plant-Based Meals" 30-day cookbook for seniors!

We hope you've enjoyed exploring the delicious flavors and health benefits of plant-based eating. Remember, adopting a plant-based diet can have numerous benefits for your health and well-being, including improved heart health, increased energy levels, and better digestion. Keep experimenting with new ingredients and recipes to continue nourishing your body and soul for years to come. Happy cooking and bon appétit!